Sok sikerrel haszmálja

Szeretettel
Magda

Okt. 20 - 2000.

THE LAZY PERSON'S GUIDE TO FITNESS

or

"I GET ALL THE
EXERCISE I NEED
WALKING AROUND
THE OFFICE"

**Charles Swencionis, Ph.D.
and E. Davis Ryan, P.T.**

Illustrations by Glenwood Lawrence

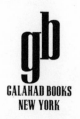

GALAHAD BOOKS
NEW YORK

TO GAE,
the treasure I found in Venice—C.S.

TO KATHY,
who has given me everything
especially Tim and Danny—E.D.R.

First Galahad Books edition published in 2000.

Galahad Books
A division of BBS Publishing Corporation
386 Park Avenue South
New York, NY 10016

Galahad Books is a registered trademark of BBS Publishing Corporation.

Published by arrangement with Barricade Books.

Library of Congress Catalog Card Number: 99-75368

ISBN: 1-57866-084-X

Designed by Cindy LaBreacht

Printed in the United States of America.

ACKNOWLEDGEMENTS

Many thanks to Sandy and Carole Stuart for making this book readable, and to Lyle for giving us the opportunity. Thanks also to Gae Rodke, Nicole Armenta, Lynn Edlen-Nezin, and Constance Bellin for their suggestions; and to Kathy Ryan, Tim and Danny Ryan, and Delores Lawrence for posing for the illustrations.

CONTENTS

INTRODUCTION

Are you part of the vast majority of Americans whose favored exercise is working the remote control? Do you get winded watching a Jane Fonda tape where, with hardly a bead of sweat, she generates more energy than a nuclear power plant? Do you drive around the supermarket parking lot for five minutes until you find a spot two feet from the door?

Face it. You're a Lazy Person. But don't feel bad. Most of us are. You know you *should* exercise. Your doctor has probably been making noises about your losing weight, getting fit—or getting diabetes, heart disease, hypertension, arthritis, or any number of other debilitating conditions.

You might want to get in shape, but all those years of inactivity are stopping you. The thought of going from having the muscle tone of a marshmallow to someone who could wear Spandex without blushing is overwhelming. It probably seems like so much work, effort, and concentration that you can't get yourself to start. And besides—and this is always the clincher—who has the time?

The answer is, plain and simple—you do, and this book will show you how. It's aimed at people who haven't exercised in years, or ever. It's designed to make exercise painless and to help you fit it into your lifestyle. It addresses the practical issues of what you can do, how, how much, how long, how often, how to have fun at it, and how to avoid getting hurt while doing it.

Moreover, it opens your eyes to the psychological roadblocks you erect that keep you from exercising. It will help motivate you, show you how to build up slowly, and how to deal with setbacks. You don't need an overdeveloped willpower to start exercising, to keep at it, and make it as much a part of your life as eating, sleeping, and smiling.

We decided to write this book because we, too, are Lazy People. By no stretch of the imagination was either of us a high-school jock. There were no four-minute miles or Olympic aspirations in our past. We liked gym class because it didn't involve algebraic equations. In many ways, we might have seemed unlikely candidates to author a book such as this. Yet, as adults, because of the twists and turns of happenstance, we came to make regular exercise an enjoyable part of our own lives, and, on a professional level, the lives of others. We sincerely believe this book can help you to do the same.

CHUCK'S STORY: I was in an auto accident twenty-three years ago and was told that I might need a hip replacement. However, with regular exercise, the hip has been largely pain free, and so far I've avoided surgery. When I cannot or do not exercise for a week or two, the pain returns and reminds me to get back on the wagon (or the treadmill). I have tried swimming, martial arts, bicycling, walking, running, stationary cycling, cross-country skiing, the stationary ski machine, and weight lifting.

At first, it was a great struggle to get myself to exercise. As I went on, I came to enjoy it. It's gotten to the point that I feel sluggish and depressed when a cold or injury keeps me from working out. Now I've come to believe that exercise is a natural part of life. Lifestyles that discourage us from moving are perverse and cause us no end of problems.

While it might be nice to believe otherwise, there is no single exercise or even single approach to exercise that is the be-all and end-all, no magic bullet, no panacea.

One thing can be said, however, with certainty—exercise should not hurt. That bromide of "no pain, no gain" is nonsense. Reaping the benefits of exercise comes from persistence, not pushing yourself into the depths of agony. I've tried different types of exercise, and there have been many times and many reasons I've fallen off the wagon. But the only times I've gotten injured or discouraged have been when I've pushed too hard and been sore the next day. Exercise is not meant to be a medieval torture. It's supposed to make you feel better—it can and will.

Professionally, I am a health psychologist, a psychologist who works with problems related to physical health, as opposed to mental health. I am associate director of the Ph.D. program in health psychology at New York's Yeshiva University. I train graduate students in health psychology and do research on weight control and cardiovascular disease. I have tried to bring some of the insights of health psychology to the book.

DAVE'S STORY: I was always interested in sports, pickup games, intramural competition, but nothing serious. And I certainly didn't "exercise" in any structured way. It wasn't part of my life. What was important to me, after a liberal arts education in the sixties and several years of uninteresting employment, was to find a fulfilling job. Working in a helping profession was appealing—and the medical field seemed to offer many opportunities, but I didn't have a clear idea of exactly what I would do in it.

Then Chuck was injured in a serious auto accident in Missoula, Montana, and I visited him there more than twenty years ago. The highlight of his day in the hospital was the visit to the physical therapist. I was impressed with how small gains in strength and increases in movement by the inch were such a source of accomplishment to him, how his progress resulted from his effort under the direction of the therapist. It hit me that this could be the challenging, satisfying profession I'd been looking for.

Physical therapy is a field that combines medical expertise, natural treatments, and the ability to offer real benefits for patients and clients. I went for it.

After obtaining a physical therapy degree from Columbia University, I worked in New York City's Presbyterian Medical Center for several years and eventually opened an office, with John Dunn, in Fort Lee, New Jersey, and then in New York City. Over the last twenty years, thousands of patients have been seen and helped in our offices.

Much of the work of a physical therapist is to evaluate a person's limitations and then to outline a course of treatment—almost always including exercise. With the advent of sports medicine, both in treating athletes and adopting a philosophy of early activity after an injury, the general public has benefited along with the pros. But it's up to the physical therapist to develop tolerable and helpful programs for people who are not motivated to exercise. Frequently patients will come to follow their exercise programs not because they should or they must, but because they want to—they enjoy exercising.

Throughout my career, I have encountered just about every type of exercise theory, new equipment, and innovative program. I have tried them all. Through trial and error, I know what does and does not work for the Lazy Person, what's going to get you going and what's going to make you throw up your hands in defeat. So forget the Marine Sergeant's Basic Training Regimen or Working Out with the Supermodel du Jour. This is the *Lazy Person's Guide to Fitness*. You may always be lazy, but that doesn't mean you can't always be fit.

This book has two parts. The first deals with the psychology of getting yourself fit. You don't have a mind set against exercise, you have a mind lock. The trick is finding the key to getting going, keeping on track—and getting yourself going again if you do stop.

The second part covers the specifics of different approaches to exercise—working out, working in, isotonic, isometric—so that you can find the types of exercises best suited to you.

HAVE FUN! You may not believe it, but you can.

EXERCISE—WHAT'S THE POINT?

In our society, children are allowed and even encouraged to be active at sports—tag, roller-skating, basketball, biking, whatever is available. Get out, get fresh air, run around, be a kid, parents urge. (Whether children do is another subject, but we'll leave that to the president's council on physical fitness.)

Once that child becomes an adult, it's a whole new ball game. Grown-ups have to do grown-up things—pay the rent or mortgage, cope with bosses and deadlines, shop for groceries and police the kitchen. Getting through the day leaves most of us with barely enough energy to climb into bed.

Yet our bodies did not evolve adapted to lives sitting behind desks, putting Pop Tarts in the toaster, driving cars two blocks to the video store. Human development between several million and twelve thousand years ago was on the plains of Africa walking, hunting, and gathering food most of the day. Our bodies were adapted to these activities and have not changed, even though our lifestyles and the demands of the world today have.

Our sedentary existence has created something of a paradox. Even though analysis of food intake per person per year in America indicates that, if anything, we eat less now than we did a few decades ago, we still gain on an average a pound a year after age twenty-five. Why? We may be eating less, but we're also doing less. The Lazy Person never walks a flight of stairs if there's an elevator.

To a degree, body weight is like a checking account: calories go in and they go out, and the balance goes up or down. Exercise spends calories; it's the prime method for making them go out. Of course, nothing is ever that simple. There is also something called the "set point." It regulates your body weight and resists being changed by adjusting metabolic rate, the rate at which your body burns food. Everyone knows someone who never stops eating but never gains a pound. That someone has a higher metabolic rate and a high set point. The Lazy Person's set point might be low now, but exercise can raise it.

With that adjustment, losing weight won't be a losing battle. You can go from being Napoleon at Waterloo to Nelson at Trafalgar. Losing weight, if you're lugging more pounds than you should, is a reason for exercising. You may want to think that only the other overweight person will suffer from hypertension, diabetes, and heart disease, and not you. Think again. Regular exercise is a tremendous weapon in the struggle against overweight.

Perhaps as important as losing pounds, regular exercise helps most people, even the Lazy Person, just feel better. We evolved walking, and an exercise as simple as that makes many people simply happier.

THE DILEMMA

Legend has it that Winston Churchill once said, "I get all the exercise I need going to the funerals of friends who have died after exercising." Harry Sahlman, an eighty-two-year-old man Dave was attempting to get up from his bed after a hip injury, had his own outlook on exercise. After graduating from Harvard in the 1920s, Harry had gone on to develop and nurture a thriving and innovative garment business. He retired by design at the age of forty-five, an extremely successful businessman. While playing golf one day with several business acquaintances, he swung and felt a sharp twinge in his back and down his leg. His immediate thought was, "Thank God, I don't have to play golf anymore."

The prospect of exercise is daunting to many people. No time, too much trouble, and fear of injury are some of the excuses given for not exercising. However, often the root of the Lazy Person's laziness is Newton's first law of motion. That's right, blame it on inertia—bodies at rest tend to stay at rest and conversely, those in motion keep moving. The standards which define life are reproduction, irritability, digestion, and motility or the ability to move.

Since the beginning of time, Man has been intrigued by movement. This fascination can be seen as early as the Cenozoic era in cave drawings, and of, course with the Greek Olympiads. At the beginning of the twentieth century, before the advent of the motion picture camera, Eadweard Muybridge devised an ingenious method for settling a bet—does a galloping horse have all four feet off the ground at once? Stretching strings attached to the shutters of many cameras across a racetrack, he created a "motion" picture and captured a horse suspended in midair as it raced down the track.

For all the studies that have been done on movement, many of us do very little of it. Children, those perpetual motion machines, become virtually motionless under certain circumstances. A recent study suggested that children burn fewer calories watching TV than sleeping. The blank stare that "Teenage Mutant Ninja Turtles" evokes is probably joined by almost total muscle inactivity. Even in sleep, most people use up some calories as they twist and turn in their beds, unlike the trancelike state TV can induce.

CHAPTER 1 SUMMARY: Our bodies evolved adapted to a life of motion, yet lifestyles now call for being sedentary. Exercise can help with weight control, hypertension, diabetes, heart disease, arthritis, depression, and other problems.

CHAPTER 2

ARE YOU READY TO EXERCISE?

H ere you are, the Lazy Person, and you want to change. So now what? There seems to be an unspannable distance between the wanting and the doing. With that in mind, James Prochaska of the University of Rhode Island and Carlo DiClemente developed a way of looking at change to help you bridge that gap.

The first thing to realize is change is not all or none. There is no magic wand that makes it happen all at once. Change comes in stages, and there are techniques that work in one stage and not in others. If you can understand which stage you're in, you can use the appropriate technique to move along.

THE SECRET OF CHANGE

The secret to making exercise a permanent part of your life is in what you do *after* you first get on the stationary bicycle or the ski machine. Don't misunderstand the meaning of exercising regularly. It's not a state where you no longer have to change. It's not like a building block that once it is put into place, it just stays there.

You shouldn't view change as an all-or-nothing thing. If you do, you will blame yourself for being weak-willed or somehow defective when you fall back into old habits and have difficulty starting again. Relapse is the rule rather than the exception. Virtually everyone falls off the wagon now and then. If you know this, you won't be so tough on yourself when it happens to you.

This is how health clubs make money. If every member came to the club three to six days a week, it would be so crowded, there would be long waiting lines at every machine. But health clubs know that most people will join, work out for some period lasting between one day and six months, and then stop.

The stages of change are cyclical, not linear. Even non-lazy people—there are some—with great bodies admit that they go through periods when they're not able to exercise. Everyone has times when they are highly motivated to change, like at New Year's; and other times when exercise is the last thing on their minds.

LEARN FROM PROBLEMS

Problems aren't necessarily bad. As Alan Marlatt of the University of Washington was first to point out, a problem doesn't have to be the first sign of failure. It can be an opportunity to learn. This perspective has created a revolution in treating addictions: drug, alcohol, gambling, overeating, and others. In a way, a sedentary life is an addiction. It's tempting to not move.

STAGES OF CHANGE

It turns out that ordinary self-changers follow the same steps that are at the core of psychotherapies. Although there are

250 to 400 types of psychotherapy, in their studies Prochaska and DiClemente were only able to identify ten frequently used processes of change.

Before you can get where you're going, you have to know where you're at. Take our Stages-of-Change Test, and see where you are now. Don't worry! The stage you are in changes all the time. You may take the test again in a week and be in a very different place. All the stages have techniques that enable you to move on, so wherever you are, you can move up.

STAGES-OF-CHANGE TEST

TRUE   FALSE

_____ _____   1. I don't want to exercise

_____ _____   2. I have thought about exercising, but no particular type appeals to me

_____ _____   3. I have thought about exercising, but I haven't made any plans to do so yet

_____ _____   4. I have thought about exercising, but I haven't actually tried it yet

_____ _____   5. I have thought about exercising, and plan to try in the next month

_____ _____   6. I have thought about exercising, and tried within the past year, but gave up

_____ _____   7. I have thought about exercising and have tried some small bits

_____ _____   8. I have actually chosen some type of exercise

_____ _____   9. I have actually started working out regularly

_____ _____ 10. I do work out regularly, but sometimes

I don't

SCORING YOUR TEST

Look at your check marks. There will be one or more questions you answered "True" to, and then some point after that where you answer "False," unless you answered "True" to question 10. The last question to which you answered "True" is your score.

If your score is 1, you're in the I Don't Want to Exercise stage.

If your score is between 2 and 5, you're in the Thinking About It stage.

If your score is between 6 and 7, you're Getting Ready.

If your score is between 8 and 9, you're in the Starting stage.

If your score is 10, you're Keeping On.

STAGE 1: "I DON'T WANT TO EXERCISE"

───────

CHUCK: _My college friend Allan didn't like to exercise. One day in gym class, we were playing crab soccer, a game where you scurry around on all fours, chest up and try to score with a huge ball. Allan was sitting on the sidelines._

"Allan!" yelled the gym teacher. "You're not playing!"

"I am playing," said Allan. "Poorly!"

───────

Allan was a classic first stager. He knew exercise was good for him, but the surgeon general could have knelt at his feet and read a report on exercise and health to him, and he still wouldn't have listened. Ignorance, denial, or having your own peculiar and skewed perspective on a situation marks this stage.

If you are at the I Don't Want to Exercise point, you might wonder what could possibly be done to get you, the Lazy Person, to budge beyond it. It's all well and good that other people might be pressuring you, but it's you that has to tie on your shoes and go out for a walk. And you don't even want to make the effort to think about it.

There are two change processes that seem to work well for people in this state of (in more ways than one) inflexibility: Gathering Information and Ranting and Whining.

Gathering Information involves finding out more about yourself and your problem. This can come externally—others observing that you don't exercise, loved ones confronting you about it—and internally—watching TV or movies about sports, reading about exercise, learning about the psychology of why people don't exercise.

Family members can try expanding a Lazy Person's knowledge with a bombardment of newspaper and magazine articles about physical activity and keeping fit, renting videos with action and sports scenes, inviting acquaintances over who actively pursue some kind of exercise and will talk about it.

If Chuck still knew Allan, he would deluge him with information about the effects of not exercising. Being sedentary increases the risks of obesity, diabetes, heart disease, arthritis, depression, and other problems.

While attempting to educate people on the dangers of not exercising can be depressing, giving people information about exercise is positive and fun. Yet despite all the good efforts of the Lazy Person's friends and relatives, the fact still remains that you don't want to exercise, so there will be very little visible effect. As Dorothy Parker said, "You can lead a horticulture, but you can't make her think." The same is true for the other process that works when you don't want to exercise.

Ranting and Whining involves giving vent to one's problem. Just talking and complaining about the problem helps. Complaining about what happened the last time you tried to exercise—"Oh, that cramp I got! I was sore for days!"—or all the things that kept you from working out—"I wanted to, but Janey had a dentist's appointment"—gets you at least thinking about exercising. It gets the wheels turning so that getting fit becomes a problem to be solved.

We all know people who like to bring drama to ordinary situations, people who like to make a big deal over little things. This penchant can be great when trying to get them to exercise. It can also be used with less drama-prone people. An individual's problems might be lack of flexibility, diabetes, or overweight, or any of the other reasons that can be helped by exercise. Talking, even complaining about them, can be used in the process leading to increased physical activity.

CHUCK: *My friend Sally, a woman in her seventies, has rheumatoid arthritis. She complains about it and dramatizes it, to point of boring her friends. But listening to Sally, letting her weep and moan over how hard it is to open jars and move around, can do her good, especially if the weeping and moaning can be turned to how hard it is to do the daily walking her* *physician has prescribed. You might think that this interminable grousing would make the problem worse, but, in fact, it gets Sally mentally processing exercise again. Thinking is the first step towards doing.*

It may seem that nothing is happening in the I Don't Want to Exercise stage, but the more Information Gathering and Ranting and Whining are used, the more their effects can accumulate.

STAGE 2: THINKING ABOUT IT

When you've reached Thinking About It, not only are you aware a problem exists, you're seriously thinking about doing something about it. This is great progress, even if you haven't made a commitment to actually start. A. Benjamin describes this stage perfectly. He was walking home when a stranger approached him and asked directions. Benjamin gave instructions, but after accepting and understanding them, the stranger went off the wrong way. Benjamin called, "You are headed in the wrong direction." The stranger answered, "Yes, I know. I am not quite ready yet."

Congratulations! By reading this book, you've at least gotten to Thinking About It, the second stage of readiness to exercise.

You're now considering the pros and cons of starting, even if you haven't quite gotten yourself to plug in the treadmill. You're at the point where you might increase your physical activity or you might decide you're not quite ready for prime time—or any other time—workouts and give it up for now.

In this stage, you know where you want to go and may even know how to get there, but you can't quite cajole yourself into following through. Gathering Information and Ranting and Whining will again be helpful along two other change processes, Role Models and Reinventing Yourself.

Role Models takes Gathering Information one step further. You want to get involved with someone who exercises, get into watching documentaries about exercise, sporting events like the Olympics, or movies with sports themes, like *Chariots of Fire*, *The Mighty Ducks*, or *Hoosiers*.

Who would be role models you respect and like? Pick some activity you enjoy, and watch a master of it. You could go to the ballet, take your kids to Disney or Sesame Street or Barney on Ice. You could get tickets to the circus and marvel at the impossible feats of the acrobats. Especially with cable, TV provides a never-ending line-up of sports. You could turn out for your local school's swimming, baseball or, soccer games.

Once you open yourself up to the possibilities, there is a huge range of physical activity you can observe. Go and watch. It will inspire you and get you to want to move that way yourself.

Reinventing Yourself is very popular these days. Japan has reinvented itself at least twice since World War II. First, as a cheap industrial imitator in the fifties. Now, as the industrial leader in its chosen fields. Politicians reinvent themselves constantly, changing parties, stealing the issues of the opposition if they're more popular. Even Richard Nixon managed to go from scandal and shame to elder statesman.

Executives, like Apple's Steve Jobs, are not above wrapping themselves in legend for others to believe.

When you reinvent yourself, you look at yourself in a different way. Have you ever played air guitar, pretending to be a rock musician? This kind of fantasy is trying out different roles for yourself. It's common in our teens and twenties, but dies out as we get older. No matter what your age, now is the time to return to the fantasy. Try imagining yourself as an athlete, or a dancer, or just someone who is really in shape.

Imagery could involve mentally picturing yourself more flexible, or thinner, or whatever else exercise could help you with. Take three minutes, sit down, lean back, close your eyes, and fantasize about downhill skiing, playing lacrosse, dancing, or anything else physical that you want to try. Just do it.

When it's over, how does it feel? If you imagine skiing, can you feel the wind? The crouch? Your body sway as you balance? Do you see the hill, the sun, snow, trees, the other skiers? Do you feel your boots, the skis, poles, your goggles, as you whiz down the trail? Is your heart beating faster, your blood pumping in your legs and arms? Can you feel the thrill in the pit of your stomach and your head when the run is through? Make it happen in your mind. The brain is extraordinarily powerful. If you think you can, you think you can, you can be the Lazy Person Who Could.

Another technique that is helpful at this stage of Thinking About It is to have fun doing something physical. It's sometimes hard to make fun things happen, but you could set the stage by going to play miniature golf or attending the company picnic softball game.

VALUES CLARIFICATION: This might be a good time to take a look at the values you hold about exercise. That is, do you believe it's good? Bad? Are certain types fun? Dreary? Is exercise only for Greek gods or goddesses, but not for you? On the following lines, write down what you feel, both positive and negative, about exercise in general and different types in specific.

1._____

2._____

3._____

4._____

5._____

6._____

Now, look at the first one. Ask yourself if it's still true for you, or if it's a holdover from some less relevant part of your past life. Do you want to change it, restate it somehow? Now look at the new version. How important a value is it to you? Rate it from 0 to 10. Go on to the other values, and do the same with them.

Look at the whole list again, from the most important to the least. Does this clarify how you relate to exercise? Does this help you see how you can approach exercise in a more useful way than you have before?

IMAGERY: Just as you imagined yourself schussing with Olympic form down the slope, you can use imagery to conjure up the benefits that will come from exercising. Think of the thing exercise could help you with that is most important to you. Could your joints be more flexible? Would you be happier ten pounds lighter? Close your eyes. Imagine yourself moving as you would like to move. Watch this in the theater of your mind for however long it interests you. When you grow bored, stop, whether five seconds have passed or ten minutes. Repeat this two or three times a day. It helps motivate you to see yourself as you would like to be.

With some goals, like movement, imagery rehearses the motor pathways so the actual movement, when tried later, is easier. With weight, imagine yourself thinner. See yourself at the beach, or doing things you feel extra weight keeps you from now. The same process works with any physical goal: picture yourself at the goal, and this image will help motivate you. Keep it up for as long as you can, hopefully until you reach your goal.

STAGE 3: GETTING READY

Getting Ready combines intending to change with making some small changes in behavior. This means more Reinventing Yourself, Values Clarification, and Imagery.

In Getting Ready, your intention and behavior crank up a notch. You may plan to begin next month or maybe you have taken some unsuccessful action in the past year. You may even be making some small attempts to exercise now.

Exercising has been on Randy W.'s To Do list for years. After watching some of the aerobic and toning shows on TV, she fantasized about looking like the women on them. Then she decided she could do those exercises. She started making tapes of the shows so she could fit them in when her schedule permitted. She is walking to work more frequently now, when she used to take a cab.

STAGE 4: STARTING

Starting—when you begin exercising on a regular basis—is what most people equate with change, overlooking the other steps that are part of the process.

This is understandable since at this fourth stage, you actually choose some type of exercise or group of activities and start working out. People can see that you've changed your behavior in order to overcome the barriers or problems that have kept you from getting fit. You appear to have gotten off the couch and thrown the shackles of the Lazy Person aside by committing time and—yes—energy.

This is the riskiest stage. Many people overdo it. Then, if they hurt or exhaust themselves, they become discouraged and drop back to I Don't Want to Exercise. If you have begun exercising and kept at it for anywhere from a day to six months, you may think you're home free. Unfortunately, not so. For true change, you must also develop skills to keep from falling back and to deal with new problems.

COMING OUT

One way to start is to announce to the world what you're about to undertake. Once you've publicly connected yourself with exercise, you have social support pushing you to keep the connection. If you stop, people will ask what happened, and you probably won't feel good about admitting failure. Your pronouncement is your debut, your Coming Out.

Coming Out is most useful in moving from preparation to action. It's all the things that make you feel free. They have very personal meanings and are different for each person. They usually involve a dramatic statement or gesture that signals a break from the past. Some people grow beards, others burn their bras. Some people leave home. Some Coming Out can be self-destructive, such as drug-taking. All have as their essence the statement made by The Who's Tommy, "I'm free!" You're declaring that the rest of your life will be different from your past. It could be as simple as buying your first pair of athletic shoes or joining a gym.

Matt had always been a sports fan but never an athlete himself. Then he began to jog. At forty-five, and a good eighty pounds overweight, he had been meaning to exercise for years. He had always liked the idea of jogging, and his knees seemed to take it well. Now, his neighbors saw him out in his sweats every morning, and he talked about it to his friends, although he tried to not bore them. He took pride in doing this for himself. He had changed the way he saw himself, adding a bit of the athlete to his self-perception. Matt has Come Out as a jogger.

If you join a gym, for example, and tell your friends and relations you have, you'll feel ashamed if you don't follow through. You'll be needled and ribbed if you don't honor your commitment. You can use this social pressure to help yourself begin to act. The same can be done with commitment to any form of exercise.

Go back to Matt, the jogger. Matt's telling his friends, neighbors, and family that he is a jogger all work to keep him jogging. They now see him a little differently, and if he stops, they will tease him about it.

BELIEVE IN YOUR ABILITY TO CHANGE

Increasing your belief in your ability and independence to change your life in key ways is mostly internal, an internal reflection of the external. What are you saying to yourself about exercise? Is it "I think I can," or is it "Maybe," or is it "I think I can't"? Whatever level of confidence you have in your ability to change, try turning it up a notch.

If you're saying "I think I can't," try saying "Maybe." If you're saying "Maybe," try "I think I can."

CHANGE YOUR WORLD

To alter your behavior, you have to believe you can do it. You have to cut yourself loose from social pressures not to change. Do you have a spouse or significant other who hates exercising as much as Churchill? Did your parents think that exercising was a waste of time? You can be your own person in this area of life without divorcing yourself from these people.

Make things easier for yourself by redecorating your world. Don't hide your ski machine under a pile of stuff in the closet. Have it out and ready to use. Seeing it can prompt you to use it. Join a gym that is on your way to or from work, or close enough to visit on your lunch hour, rather than one you have to make an effort to get to.

REWARD YOURSELF

There is nothing like a little positive reinforcement in the Starting stage. Promise yourself a treat if you exercise today. Obviously, if you're trying to lose weight, don't make the reward food. Call a friend you haven't talked to in a while, or get tickets to something you would like to see. Chuck incorporates his reward with his exercising. He likes to watch videotapes while on the ski machine or stationary bicycle. When he rides a real bicycle, the scenery unfolding around him is a reward.

HELPING RELATIONSHIPS

Helping relationships can also be valuable at this stage. This can range from being open and trusting about trying to exercise with someone who cares, or discussing problems you feel prevent you from exercising with a psychotherapist. This could be a therapist you've seen before or a new relationship with a health or sports psychologist. You don't need to be crazy to see a psychotherapist. They can be helpful for anyone trying to make a change. Health and sports psychologists are especially trained to help people make changes in their habits and behavior related to their bodies.

Let's say you're trying to start exercising, and your spouse keeps scheduling other activities for the time you've slotted for your workout. You start to get the message that he or she doesn't want you to exercise. While your relationship is paramount, you shouldn't have to choose. Talking this over with someone impartial could be helpful.

STAGE 5: KEEPING ON

You've gotten to Keeping On when you can successfully overcome new obstacles that can get in the way and not lose the gains you've made in the Starting stage.

Mastering this stage is crucial if exercising is to be an integral part of the rest of your life. It's easy to start exercising: the exercise equipment in closets, basements, and classified ads, and the gym memberships that are not used attest to the difficulty of staying with it.

The techniques for Keeping On are the sum of all the techniques that got you this far. Use whatever tricks work for you. It doesn't matter if they're different from the ones that help your best friend or Cindy Crawford. Although don't forget that you can learn from what works for other people and especially from what is interfering with exercise for you right now.

Remember what we said earlier: the stages of change are cyclical, or like a spiral. You may work yourself all the way up to Keeping On, but then you get sick or injured, or take a trip, or otherwise get distracted.

You may not be in Keeping On anymore, or even in Starting. You may have dropped all the way back to Thinking About It or even I Don't Want to Exercise. Nothing magical about reaching Keeping On will keep you there. If you find yourself at some lower level, you have to use the techniques appropriate to that level to climb back up. Then you may have to use bits of them to keep on Keeping On.

Joe and Betty have difficulty knowing exactly how much of the truth to tell each other. They have a very intimate relationship and value each other's opinion highly. A cutting remark from one will really hurt the other and be remembered for a long time. For years Joe was a slug, but Betty couldn't tell him. She was afraid that telling him he had become a couch potato would become a thorn in their relationship.

In addition, Betty was afraid if Joe got back in shape, he would become attractive to other women, and she might have to compete for his attention or lose him. At the same time, he was becoming less attractive to her.

Finally Joe's declining appeal overwhelmed Betty's insecurity. She told him he had become a slug. Initially Joe was stunned and hurt. After nursing his hurt feelings for a while, he recovered, admitting he had already reached the same conclusion himself. He knew he was out of shape and had occasionally thought about getting some exercise. Hearing it from Betty spurred Joe to action. He got his old bicycle tuned up and started riding on weekends. Then he bought an expensive stationary bike that gave him complicated uphill and downhill programs to use inside on bad weather days.

Did any of that sound familiar to you? Are you having difficulties with your spouse or significant other? Is that getting you depressed or lowering your self-image to the point you're not interested in your appearance? Would exercise give you some strength and independence from any of these problems—the relationship, depression, or your self-esteem? Or do you have to work on it first before you can motivate yourself to exercise?

A note of caution, if you've made it to adulthood without exercising regularly, talk to your physician. Let him or her know you plan to engage in mild to moderate aerobic exercise, raising your heart rate to between 60 and 80 percent of capacity. Most likely, your physician will approve, unless you have a chronic condition that restricts the kinds of exercise you can do safely, in which case your doctor will advise you about this.

For most people, however, and most conditions, some type of exercise is just what your doctor would order.

This table will help you see the Stages of Change together with what they mean for your exercise program: which change techniques work best at each stage.

STAGES OF CHANGE	WHAT THIS MEANS FOR YOUR EXERCISE PROGRAM: A TOOLBOX OF THE BEST TECHNIQUES FOR EACH STAGE
I Don't Want To Exercise	Get More Information About Exercise
Talk About Exercise	Complain About How Hard It Is and How Much You Hate It Rant and Whine

Thinking About It	Consider Pros and Cons
	Get More Information
	Complain, Rant and Whine
	Watch Role Models
	Reinvent Yourself as an Athlete or as Someone In Shape
	Imagine Yourself Exercising
	Have Fun Doing Something Physical
	Clarify Values About Exercise

Getting Ready	Reinvent Yourself
	See Exercise as Part of Your Life
	Clarify Values About Exercise
	Imagine Yourself Exercising

Starting	Come Out
	Believe in Your Ability to Change
	Reward Yourself
	Use Helping Relationships
	Change Your World
	Exercise Instead of Doing Something Else
	Imagery

Keeping On	Everything From Earlier Stages That Works for You
	Learn From Problems (see Chapter 5)

CHAPTER 2 SUMMARY: The stages of readiness to change include I Don't Want to Exercise, I'm Not Ready Yet, Getting Ready, Starting, and Keeping On. The stages of change are not linear but cyclical. Recognizing what stage you're in can help you progress. I Don't Want to Exercise is helped most by techniques of Gathering Information and Ranting and Whining. These techniques are also helpful in I'm Not Ready Yet, and so are Role Models and Reinventing Yourself. Getting Ready is helped by Reinventing Yourself. Starting is encouraged by Coming Out, Choosing, Commitment to Act, Increasing Belief in Your Ability and Autonomy to Change, Changing Your World, and Rewards. Keeping On is promoted by all the techniques you have used to get this far, as well as by realizing that each slip is an opportunity for learning.

CHAPTER 3

BUILDING EXERCISE INTO YOUR LIFE

WORKING OUT VERSUS WORKING IN

Does "exercise" conjure up visions of muscled fitness freaks clad in Spandex and Wesson Oil, exhorting viewers of some obscure cable channel to FEEL THAT BURN? You're a Lazy Person. Probably the only thing you've ever felt like burning is a log in your fireplace.

Don't be discouraged by these TV androids. Take heart in knowing that there are two broad approaches to exercise: 1) you can spend some time each day or week at some specific training (working out), or, 2) you can take the stairs and park far from your destination so that you walk more (working in). You can choose either or both approaches, but some people have a lifestyle that lends itself more easily to one or the other.

BOTH HAVE THEIR ADVANTAGES

The advantage of the gym/spa/home gym is that if you're pressed for time, you don't have to worry about choosing between taking the stairs or being on time for an appointment. You don't have to think about exercise constantly but only during your exercise time. You select set times each week for regular workouts. Once exercising is committed to your schedule, you don't have to think about it beyond that. Another plus to this route is being able to precisely target your workouts to your goals.

If you approach exercise by working it into your daily life (walking, climbing stairs), you don't have to change your self-concept to that of an exerciser. Another benefit is that you don't have to spend money on a gym or equipment. And you don't have to schedule anything additional into a busy life.

WORKING OUT

You may be a Lazy Person, but you're also a busy one. It's hard to find time to exercise. The last thing you need is another task to squeeze into your already hectic day, one more item on your schedule to add to your stress. Right? Wrong! Exercise will give you more energy for the other things in your life. You'll be less stressed, less frazzled, more able to concentrate, better able to sleep.

Moreover, working out doesn't have to be an onerous, boring chore. Many people find they can read while they exercise on a stationary bike or stair-climbing machine. Chuck frequently reads journal articles, student papers, and other work-related material on the exercise bicycle. In fact, he finds he's more likely to spend an uninterrupted period of time reading during exercise than at home with his children clamoring for his attention or in the office with the phone ringing.

In many ways, exercise is a form of meditation. Because it is repetitive, it narrows your focus of attention, and when your attention drifts, it must be brought back. At the beginning of an exercise session, Chuck will ask himself one question, such as how to organize this section of this book. Then he'll find that possibilities float in and out of his head. By the end of the session, he's made some progress. Like meditation, the focus of exercise helps keep extraneous ideas and pressures out of your mind.

WORKING IN

You may not want to set aside a particular time to do something different from your regular life called "exercise." Do you become ill when people prattle on about their exercise routines? Do presidents and political candidates who jog make you wish there were a third party?

The human body didn't evolve with access to a gym. Our hunter-gatherer ancestors spent much of their time walking and climbing, and this may suit you. Climbing stairs is possible in modern society, but more time is spent complaining about why the elevator is so slow than actually using the stairs. Many people in Chuck's office building take the elevator one floor, while others walk up thirteen flights.

Climbing stairs strengthens the quadriceps muscles, the muscles on the front of the thigh, builds cardiovascular endurance, and can function as aerobic exercise. The trick to climbing stairs is to check your heart rate, keep it in the range you want, and keep track of how many minutes you spend at it each day.

If stair climbing doesn't appeal to you, try walking, possibly the best exercise. The human body was designed for it, and there are lots of places to do it. It requires no special equipment or training. Almost anyone can walk. If you have a dog, take him for an extra trot outside, or extend your usual route. It's good for you and the pooch.

Walking outside when the weather is fine is best, but the world is not always cooperative. In bad weather, many shopping malls don't mind if people use their climate-controlled environment for walking. In fact, some malls even have formal "Mall Walkers" clubs that meet an hour or so before opening.

City dwellers have plenty of opportunities to walk. If you take public transportation, get off one train stop or several bus stops early and walk to your destination. Going to the store can often be done on foot. As with stair climbing, keep track of the time so you know how long you've gone.

Contrary to those who tell us we must get our heart rate up to 65 percent of capacity to gain some benefit from walking, any exercise is better than none, and the more the better, up to a point. If you were close to that point, you would be reading *Power Lifting* or *Power Running* and not *The Lazy Person's Guide to Fitness*. However, getting your heart rate up to 60 percent or 65 percent of capacity will provide additional aerobic benefit for your cardiovascular system and for weight control.

To measure your heart rate, put the index and middle fingers of one hand on the wrist of the other arm just below the base of the thumb and inside the bone of the wrist. You should feel your pulse. If you don't get a clear pulse, try two other places. One is where the artery brings blood into the head. You can find that on either side of your neck, outside the windpipe, about three fingers down from the jaw. The other place to take your heart rate is right over your heart.

Using a watch with a second hand, count the number of beats in six seconds and then multiply by ten to get your heart rate in beats per minute.

If you've never exercised or haven't for a long time, you may be able to attain this heart rate (see table on 60 percent to 80 percent of capacity) by ordinary walking. But as you get into better shape, you may not. You may have to adopt some of the principles of racewalking if you want to get aerobic benefits.

TARGET HEART RATES BY AGE

AGE	60% OF CAPACITY	80% OF CAPACITY
20	120	160
25	195	156
30	114	152
35	111	148
40	108	144
45	105	140
50	102	136
55	99	132
60	96	128
65	93	124
70	90	120
75	87	116
80	84	112
85	81	108

HEALTHWALKING

Healthwalking is a variation on how you normally walk. Try this first, and when you're comfortable with it, you may want to move up to racewalking. Even if you don't, healthwalking can make ordinary walking more comfortable and beneficial.

In healthwalking, you bend the knee a bit as the front foot touches the ground, keeping it bent through most of your stride, while your arms swing opposite to your legs. You must stand tall, be relaxed, and balance equally on your feet. Your head should be level, not dropped forward or down, nor pointing up in the air. Don't slump into your hips. Keep your ribs lifted to allow room to breathe. Shoulders should be relaxed and low, not up around your ears.

Keep this posture as you walk. Your foot should land heel first, roll forward, and push off from the toes. Keep your weight balanced directly over your hips, and don't let your head bounce or bob. Use your abdominal muscles, not your back muscles, to support your torso.

How long to make each stride depends on your leg strength, flexibility, and general strength, as well as leg length. Your stride may lengthen as you put time into walking.

Let your whole arm swing naturally, in a fairly straight arc from the shoulder. The faster you walk, or the steeper the hill, the more your arms should swing to balance your legs. Keep your arms close in to your sides. Never forget to breathe. (See figure 1.)

RACEWALKING

Racewalking involves keeping one foot on the ground at all times and having the weight-bearing leg straight at the knee

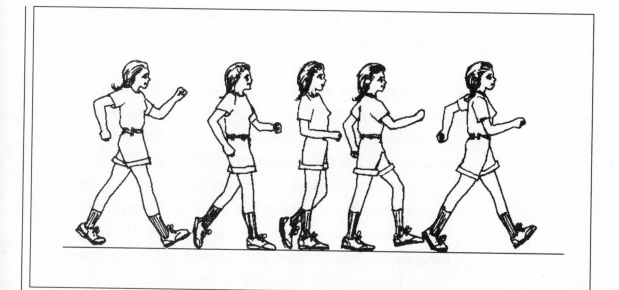

FIGURE 1

when that leg is directly under the body. You shouldn't lose contact with the ground or allow the knee to bend when it's directly under the body. The closer you adhere to these two directions, the faster you can racewalk and the more you're protected from impact with the ground.

Always keep your arms bent at a 90-degree angle at the elbow while racewalking. Swing your arms in this position from your shoulders, emphasizing the part of the swing behind the body. Keep your arms close to your sides, and don't punch them forwards.

Body posture should be the same as in healthwalking. If you slump, you'll have difficulty breathing and moving flexibly. Your whole body should lean forward slightly at an angle from the feet.

Each arm swings to counterbalance the opposite leg. Keep the two sides as symmetrical as possible. Your heel touches the ground first. You roll through the middle and outer part of your foot, and push off with the outer, small toes. If your shins are sore after a walk, you're not letting the toes drop down after the push off to let the shin muscles rest.

If your leg is almost straight as soon as your heel touches the ground, it will be easy to make it completely straight by the time it's directly under you. This may seem unnatural at first, but it becomes comfortable with practice.

To accentuate the pumping action of the arms and add to the aerobic effect, you may wish to hold or wrap around your wrists light, one-to-three-pound, weights. However, as a Lazy Person starting out, you should be able to achieve adequate heart rate without adding weights. In fact, racewalking comes close to working out, rather than working in, but its principles are useful. (See figure 1.)

SHOES

If walking or climbing stairs is going to be your sport, you need comfortable shoes. Flat shoes, wide enough in the front to allow some spreading and preferably with a rubber sole, will do, especially if you're climbing stairs at work. Many people wear athletic shoes for their commute and carry or keep more formal shoes for the office or place of business.

If you exercise in high heels or tight shoes or shoes that rub your heels, you'll be very, very sorry. Very sorry. Exercising isn't the time to worry about looking good. Just remember, it won't be long before you're looking good because you're exercising.

TAKE AN EXERCISE BREAK

CHUCK: *As I am writing this, I come to points where I haven't thought out what comes next, or a transition, or am not happy with what I've written. Sometimes I'll just sit at the computer and think, but once or twice an hour, I get up and walk around. I might climb several flights of stairs, or go to the kitchen for a snack or drink, or walk the dog. A walk can help reorganize thoughts, provide a fresh insight, or a different perspective. Ten three-minute exercise breaks add up to thirty minutes of exercise in a day.*

CHAPTER 3 SUMMARY: Build your exercise plan so that it fits into your life as easily as possible. You can use a general strategy of working out, picking a gym or other time and place when and where you exercise, and just scheduling it. Or you can plan a strategy of working in, adding more movement to your daily routine by taking the stairs instead of the elevator, walking more, and taking exercise breaks. Contrary to what many exercise gurus have said, there is no one best exercise, and even getting your heart rate to 60 percent of your maximum provides cardiovascular benefits.

CHAPTER 4

THE SECRET OF THE LAZY PERSON'S GUIDE TO FITNESS

*T*he *Lazy Person's Guide to Fitness* aims to get you exercising without pain or fatigue. As you become experienced and see the benefits, exercise will become fun. The secret is to start gradually—and build gradually.

Whether you chose Working Out or Working In, or any combination, you should follow this plan. Start with one minute the first day. You didn't misread that. ONE MINUTE. Add half a minute the second day and each subsequent day, until you get to your goal. Does this seem slow? It is. You may feel that you're going *too* slowly. You're not. This is the essence, the secret of the Lazy Person's approach to fitness.

"Slow" is the key word. Why? The answer is simple. If your body is not used to exercise, it needs time to acclimate. Exercise causes your body to change. Your heart beats faster, it pumps more blood, your blood pressure goes up, more blood is delivered to the muscles and to your brain per minute. The muscles swell from this, and the exertion causes small tears in them.

In between exercise times, your heart beats more slowly, your blood pressure is lower, and your metabolism increases compared to before you began your exercise program. The swelling in the muscles resolves, and the small tears heal.

Regular repetition causes these changes to progress, and as the small tears heal, the muscle increases in strength. You lose fat and build muscle.

However, there is a cost if you push too hard and too fast. Arnold Schwarzenegger and Jane Fonda didn't build their bodies without pain. When you push your workout to beyond what your body can handle, it will hurt.

The seventies gave us that "go for the burn," while in the eighties we had "no pain, no gain." The misguided rehabilitation version of this is, "no squeal, no heal"—you've got to feel bad before you get better. This slogan, that pain is necessary for building fitness, is totally false. Building half a minute per day pushes the body just hard enough to condition without pain or fatigue. The swelling and little tears will be small enough so that they will heal without your really noticing. If you "burn" and are in pain, you're causing tissue damage which takes time to heal.

OOPS—I MISSED A DAY!

What happens when you miss a day? Nothing. If you're increasing your exercise time by a half minute daily, skipping a day isn't a cause for concern. In fact, you can go three days without exercising and take up exactly where you left off. However, once you take four or more days off, your body will have lost some of its conditioning, and you'll need to make an adjustment to your exercise time. Subtract a half minute for each day beyond three that you've missed, and go from there.

What happens if you get sick or injured? If you're sick with a bacterial or viral infection, your body needs extra energy to fight the infection and repair itself. It doesn't need the additional stress of exercise. However, there will come a time when the symptoms have gone from acute to recovering, when you're well past any fever. At that point, you can consider returning to exercise. If exercise makes any symptoms worse, if it makes your heart beat faster than your experience indicates it should, if you feel faint or get a headache, if you get short of breath or have pain rather than brief, mild discomfort, then you returned too early.

Use the formula of subtracting one half minute per day beyond three to determine how many minutes to exercise the first day of return, and then build up by a half minute per day again.

Injuries are tricky. Some necessitate no exercise, and others can be worked around. For example, Chuck frequently has difficulties with his knee, the result of his old Montana accident. When he does, he switches to exercises that do not bother it.

Okay, Lazy Person, this is something you've always wanted to hear. In general, *never do any exercise that hurts.* If you have questions about particular injuries, ask your doctor or physical therapist.

WHAT DO YOU WANT?

Goals for an exercise program are as different as the people who exercise. Some people want to look better. Others wish to treat health problems. Or have you been feeling sluggish and not liking what you see in the mirror. (Who is that Fat Person, anyway?) You might be tired of having sand kicked in your face at the beach and want to be stronger. Or maybe you've seen actuarial charts for the average couch potato and hope to increase your chances of living longer. Once you've decided what it is that you want to achieve, there is a menu of exercises to choose from to help you reach your goals.

Keep in mind—should you feel overwhelmed by the concept of getting fit—any exercise is better than none. You will not get into shape overnight, but you can feel and look better little by little. Different types and amounts of exercise produce different effects and will help you set goals.

LOSING WEIGHT

Lots of people want to lose weight. It may be to look better, or feel better, or out of concern for their health. Of course, eating low-fat foods, lots of fruits, vegetables, grains, and beans is helpful. The "Food Pyramid" promoted by the U.S. Department of Agriculture reflects a low-fat diet that will help take off excess weight and improve health. (See figure 2.)

This diagram shows the base of the pyramid, what people should eat most, as six to eleven servings per day of bread, cereal, rice, and pasta, the grain group. The next level of the pyramid, the vegetable and fruit groups, is a little narrower, with three to five servings of vegetables, and two to four servings of fruit. Up another step at the dairy and protein groups, only two to three servings of low-fat milk, yogurt, and cheese, and two to three servings of lean meat, poultry, fish, dry beans, eggs, and nuts are suggested. At the tiniest point of the pyramid is fats, oils, and sweets, which should be eaten sparingly.

Serving size is also important. You shouldn't fudge—if you'll excuse the expression—here. One serving of bread is

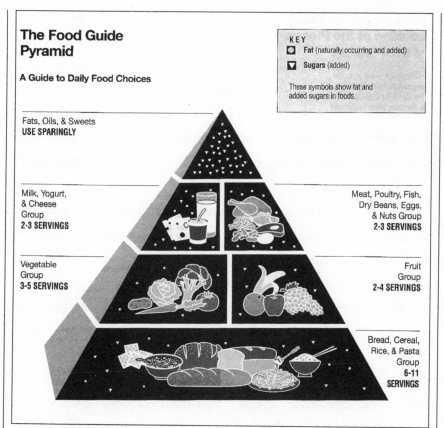

The Food Guide Pyramid

A Guide to Daily Food Choices

KEY
◯ Fat (naturally occurring and added)
▽ Sugars (added)

These symbols show fat and added sugars in foods.

Fats, Oils, & Sweets
USE SPARINGLY

Milk, Yogurt, & Cheese Group
2-3 SERVINGS

Meat, Poultry, Fish, Dry Beans, Eggs, & Nuts Group
2-3 SERVINGS

Vegetable Group
3-5 SERVINGS

Fruit Group
2-4 SERVINGS

Bread, Cereal, Rice, & Pasta Group
6-11 SERVINGS

FIGURE 2

one slice, not one loaf. Most people need no more protein each day than a single serving of lean meat, poultry, or fish about the size of a deck of cards. Most Americans eat far more protein than this and most of it with a lot of fat attached.

Besides eating right, exercise can help you lose weight, with aerobic exercise being the most helpful. Yoga, stretching, and weight training will help other problems but won't do much in your battle with the bulge.

Aerobics entails the smooth and rhythmic exercising of your major muscle groups, especially your legs and buttocks, and if possible, also your arms. You must move at a speed fast enough to reach at least 60 percent of your maximum heart rate (see table on page 35) and yet not so fast that you cannot carry on a conversation. You mustn't exercise so hard that you become short of breath.

Start timing your aerobic exercise (sixty seconds the first day, add thirty seconds each subsequent day) when you reach your target heart rate. More details about aerobic exercise are in Chapter 10.

Any aerobic exercise performed regularly will help you lose weight. That's the good news. The bad news is exercise won't do it alone. You won't get rid of those extra pounds unless you're also careful about what you eat.

It's also important not to starve yourself. Any weight loss program should be set up so that you eat a balanced, nutritious diet of at least 1,200 calories per day. Falling below this, the body responds as if it's coming into a period of famine. The metabolic rate drops, you feel slowed down and depressed, and you don't achieve sustainable weight loss.

What we mean by sustainable weight loss is no more than 1 percent of body weight per week: that translates to 2 pounds for a 200-pound person, 1 1/2 pounds for a 150-pound person, 3 pounds for a 300-pound person.

Don't forget, the average American gains one pound a year after age twenty-five. If you can maintain your weight and not gain this pound per year, it's a victory in itself.

If you aren't satisfied with maintaining your weight and want to lose ten, fifteen pounds or more, what is the optimum amount of exercise to help you do that? Hold onto your running shoes: you may be surprised. We stand by our statement that *any* amount of regular aerobic exercise will help you lose weight. However, how much weight you lose and how fast you lose it depends on how much you exercise.

If you really want to have some impact on weight, you should exercise at least twenty minutes, three times a week. If you want to have more effect, exercise thirty to sixty minutes, five or six times a week.

These are potential goals. Exercise is something you want to fit into your life, not something you want to fit your life into. If ten minutes twice a week is all you can do, in the long run, you're better off doing that rather than nothing. You're also less likely to hurt yourself at that level. Don't push yourself beyond a goal you can live with. If you find you can't live with it, change it. *But don't give up.*

Whatever goal you set, remember the Lazy Person's secret. Build by only a half minute per day. Start counting your exercise time from when your heart rate reaches 60 percent of your capacity. Never let it get beyond 80 percent of capacity, or to where your breathing so hard you can't carry on a conversation.

LIVING LONGER

Ralph Paffenbarger, an epidemiologist at Stanford University, has done a series of studies relating exercise and longevity. He has followed 10,269 alumni of Harvard College since 1962. Men who were quite sedentary, expending less than 2,000 calories per week in all their activity, had a 25 percent higher risk of death at the same age than more active men. Men who didn't engage in moderately vigorous sports activity, such as swimming, tennis, squash, racquetball, handball, jogging, or running, had a 44 percent higher risk of death at the same age than those who did.

Ah, you say, perhaps the men who exercised more were healthier to begin with. Paffenbarger also looked at estimates of the years added to alumni's lives who adopted exercise later in life. The average amount of life-span added to the entire group of men from 45 to 84 years of age was an additional 0.72 year for those taking up moderately vigorous sports. The amount of lifespan added varied from .85 year for those 45 to 54, .73 year for those 55 to 64, .48 year for those 65 to 74, and .18 year for those 75 to 84.

Another way to look at this is that a half hour of exercise buys you about an extra hour of life.

GETTING STRONGER AND FIRMER

You don't have to be an aspiring Mr. or Ms. Muscle Beach to want to increase muscle strength and tone. There are many other reasons why you would want to get stronger and firmer. Without exercise, we lose muscle strength, bulk, and tone as we age. If body weight stays the same or goes up, body composition shifts more towards fatness. What looked firm and compact at twenty has the consistency of mashed potatoes at fifty.

Pain from osteoarthritis or rheumatoid arthritis can often be reduced by increasing the strength and tone of the major muscles surrounding the joint. For example, hip pain can be reduced by increasing the strength and tone of the quadriceps (the major muscle on the front of the thigh) and the muscles that move your leg back (buttocks), in (adductor), and out (abductor).

Back pain can often be alleviated by working on the abdominal muscles.

Weight training can reverse the loss of strength and tone at any age. A study of people in their seventies and eighties showed that mild weight training caused them to increase strength, muscle mass, and tone.

HOW DO YOU TONE?

Basically to tone, you lift, push, or pull until the muscle is tired. This stimulates it to adapt to a higher level of use: it increases in strength and tone as it recovers. This can be accomplished by weight training, isometrics, or some combination of both.

We go into details on strengthening and increasing tone in the second half of the book.

MOVING MORE EASILY

The more you move, as long as you don't do anything that hurts, the more you increase flexibility and ease of movement. When you wake up in the morning, your joints are stiff. As you go through your morning preparations, they loosen and free themselves.

A friend of Chuck's interviewed Pablo Casals, the famous cellist, when he was ninety years old and still actively giving concerts. The whole time they spoke, Casals was opening and closing his hands. "It keeps the arthritis away," he said, and he was very impressive proof of that.

"Use it or lose it" is the way joints work. Processes of strengthening, stretching, and every combination of them have some benefit. This can be pursued by formal exercises, sports, dancing, walking, or any other activity that gets you moving.

Is all moving the same? Of course not. But the kinds of moving we really enjoy, that we'll keep doing for the long run, are better than the optimal exercise that we won't do. This is true up to the point of pain. If you enjoy some activity such as tennis or racquetball, but it hurts, you may have to compromise on some less enjoyable but less harmful sport.

Stretching, very important if done correctly, increases the range a joint can move through without pain. The correct way to stretch is to take the joint to the limit it can move without pain and hold it there for at least thirty seconds. Do not bounce. Hold the position steadily and push a little farther during the thirty seconds if you find you can without pain. Bouncing activates a reflex which keeps the muscle from relaxing enough to stretch as far as it can.

Strengthening improves flexibility and ease of movement by increasing the tone of muscles directly surrounding the joint. Added muscle support takes some of the stress from the joint. Flexibility and ease of movement improve through weight training, isometrics, aerobic exercise, sports, dancing, or any other activity that builds muscle tone.

SPOT REDUCING AND CELLULITE

Everyone's body is different. Yet we all have ideals we dream about: bodies that we would like to have and bodies of others that we find attractive. Many women have been influenced by a Barbie-doll ideal and want an impossibly freakish body like hers: very tall and slender, with large breasts that do not sag, and slim, boyish hips and thighs. If you have a genetic propensity to accumulate fat in your hips and thighs, wish all you want. You'll never look like Barbie. But really, who cares? There's something plastic about her, anyway.

When we lose weight, we lose it all over. The face, arms, trunk, buttocks, hips, thighs, and everywhere else lose some fat. Human body fat, in consistency, is like butter. Take a pound of butter, and hold it against your belly. It's substantial. If you can, hold five pounds against yourself. It's quite an impressive amount of bulk. When you lose one pound or five pounds, it's equivalent to those pounds of butter held against your midsection.

Cellulite is those lumpy accumulations of fat just below the skin. If we could spot reduce, almost everyone would get rid of them first. But there is no such thing as spot reducing.

There are two things you *can* do to combat cellulite. First, control your weight through regular aerobic exercise and a low-fat diet. Second, tone the muscles in the cellulite areas. This means doing aerobic exercise that works those muscles and doing high-repetition (eighteen or more) weight training with light weights.

Avoid heavy weights. They will build strength and bulk, which you don't want in cellulite areas. If you have a tendency to develop "thunder thighs," this may mean you have as much a propensity to build muscle as fat in your thighs. The same may apply to other cellulite areas.

Recently creams containing aminophylline have shown promise in reducing cellulite. It's too early to be certain, but these may act on fat metabolism and reduce cellulite. Miracles, after all, can happen.

HIGH BLOOD PRESSURE, CHOLESTEROL, AND DIABETES

These conditions can be significantly improved by controlling weight through regular aerobic exercise and low-fat diet. Many lay people (and some physicians) have thought that in order to treat these problems with weight reduction, patients had to attain "ideal body weight" as specified by the Metropolitan Life Insurance tables. This, unfortunately, has proved to be an unattainable goal for most people, and only briefly attainable for others, leading to regaining weight, frustration, and discarding the weight-control strategy.

You don't have to be at that "perfect" Metropolitan Life Insurance weight to lower your high blood pressure and cholesterol count and help control diabetes. Recent research has shown that weight loss of ten to fifteen pounds can be as effective as many drugs for treating these problems. In many cases, the condition improves enough with weight control to withdraw from drug treatment altogether. Even when it doesn't, often the drug dosage can be much reduced.

FEELING GOOD

Regular exercise has been shown in a number of studies to increase a person's sense of well-being as well as decrease depression and anxiety. Depression, in particular, can be improved by exercise treatment. The most effective treatments for depression are cognitive therapy and the careful administration of drugs such as Prozac and Zoloft.

———————————

James has been in and out of treatment for depression for years. At thirty-six, he has a stable job and a stable marriage, but sometimes he is so depressed, he can't get out of bed. He saw a cognitive therapist when he felt really blue and has had good results with medication. Lately, he has begun a regular program of running and finds that he feels down much less than he used to. The depression is not gone, but like therapy and medication, exercise helps.

———————————

Making a change in one's routine helps depression. If untreated, depression often tends to get better. Exercise may have this sort of nonspecific effect on the problem. But it's also quite possible that we're returning to the body something it needs. If we evolved walking and running on the plains of Africa, it seems logical that our bodies need something like the exercise we evolved doing.

Whether this is an effect of blood being pumped to all the nooks and crannies of the brain and other parts of the body, bringing oxygen and carrying away waste, or some effect of endorphins or other naturally manufactured chemicals in the body, no one knows. But it does seem to work.

It has been mostly the effect of aerobic exercise on mood that has been studied. It's clear that this kind of exercise will help mood, but we don't know whether other types will.

COMING BACK FROM HEART DISEASE

The approach to regular, aerobic conditioning in *The Lazy Person's Guide to Fitness* will help in rehabilitation from coronary heart disease (myocardial infarction or heart attack, or angina pectoris) or for prevention of coronary heart disease. Pick one or more types of aerobic activity: walking, exercise bicycle, ski machine, actual bicycling, running, etc. Exercise to get your heart rate up to 60 percent of capacity. Keep it there the first day for 60 seconds, and add 30 seconds a day, until you get to your goal.

Walter, at sixty-six, suffered an uncomplicated heart attack and then had bypass surgery. Although he had been active all his life, his doctor ordered him to give up the heavy lifting he did at his job and to adopt a program of walking. Over a period of eighteen weeks, he worked up gradually from walking half a mile to walking four miles in an hour, three times a week.

The goal in rehabilitation from a heart attack and prevention of another one should be to hold the heart rate at 60 to 65 percent of capacity for 45 minutes at a time, 5 times per week. Don't be too aggressive in getting to this level. Stay with the Lazy Person's gradual method. Do not exercise at 75 or 80 percent of capacity to try to get into shape faster. You're not in a contest; you're not going for bragging rights. You're aiming for better health and a longer life.

Terence Kavanagh, of the Toronto Rehabilitation Center, which specializes in postcoronary exercise programs, has cardiac rehabilitation patients run marathons. If he's your cardiologist, go ahead. Otherwise, follow your own cardiologist's recommendations.

The directions here are for people who have uncomplicated coronary heart disease or angina. For those who have different or more complicated heart conditions, it's especially important to closely adhere to the instructions of your own doctor who is familiar with your own case.

People with cardiac problems must pay close attention to what their bodies are telling them. (Actually, that holds true for everyone.) Target rates are fine. They're something to aim for—reaching that desired percentage of capacity, for instance. But there is also something called the symptom rate—this is how fast your heart is beating when you feel something going wrong. If you have pain in your chest or arms, profuse sweating, dizziness, severe shortness of breath, or any other indication that you are overdoing it, you should stop exercising and rest.

Don't start exercising again until you see your doctor. You'll need to describe what happened and have a thorough cardiac evaluation. The physician will then be able to tell you how much and how hard to exercise. With cardiac testing, the target heart rate for exercise can be much more accurate that the formula of 220 minus age times 65 percent. If you have a cardiac condition, you should not have your heart rate increase by more than 20 to 30 beats over your resting level, unless you and your physician have decided on a different target heart rate during exercise.

The resting level is your heart rate after sitting comfortably for ten or fifteen minutes. So if your resting rate is seventy beats per minute, and you have a cardiac problem, you should keep your heart rate below one hundred when exercising unless you have consulted with a physician.

OH, MY ACHING BACK!

You may think you know why your back hurts—shoveling out your driveway for the fifteenth time in the season, forgetting to tell your body you were faking right and going left while driving the lane, bending at the waist to hoist a crying toddler to your comforting shoulder. And you may think time is on your side, and a few leg lifts here and stretches there will heal your aching back. Don't bet your kid's college tuition on it.

The source of back pain should be carefully diagnosed before attempting to treat it with exercise. You should see a physician who may refer you to a physical therapist. The therapist can teach you specific and effective exercises for back pain relief. In many cases these are aimed at strengthening the back, abdomen, and sides. Stronger muscles in those areas can better help support the back and take some of the strain off the spine.

CAN I IMPROVE MY TENNIS?

Forty years ago, few athletes trained with weights in addition to practicing the nuts and bolts of their particular sport. Today weight training is more the rule than the exception.

If you want to improve that backhand or smash that overhead lob on the tennis court, you would do well to build up one set of muscles and increase flexibility in certain joints. If your goal is to bowl more than one frame without your arm falling off, then you're looking at different muscles and joints.

It's difficult to generalize about improving your game in a specific sport, and you may wish to consult a coach or physical therapist. However, performance and enjoyment of almost any sport can be enhanced by regular aerobic exercise, and often by building strength and flexibility.

JUST DOING IT

Find a time of day that you can regularly work out. Some people like exercising first thing in the morning, before breakfast. Others prefer lunchtime and have a quick bite on the way back to work or eat at their desk. Chuck likes the end of the workday best, when he can read, or think about something for tomorrow, and begin the transition to home.

Some people are able to make exercising a priority. They don't have a set time but rather make time in their daily schedule as they go along. Others must have the discipline of having their workout time chiseled in stone. If it's five o'clock, it must be treadmill time. Whenever you exercise, try to make a time for it every day. You will not actually work out seven days a week, no one should. But having a regular time helps you to get exercise as many days as possible.

If you have an awful day, you'll not get a chance. If you have a terrible week, and instead of exercising six times, you only exercise three, that's OK. Skipping workouts doesn't make you a Bad Person. But do the best you can under the circumstances.

Try to exercise six days a week. If you have a particularly busy day, you won't be able to, but you still may be able to get in three to five days in the week. No one should do the same exercise all the time. It doesn't give the body a chance to recover. On one day walk, on another try the cross-country skiing machine. Mix it up—it's also better for you psychologically because the the boredom factor is decreased.

But keep in mind that three days of exercise provide significantly greater benefits than one or two. Five or six have significantly greater benefits for weight control than four or fewer. But whatever you do, just do something.

CHAPTER 4 SUMMARY: The secret of *The Lazy Person's Guide to Fitness* is to start with very little exercise, about a minute the first day and to increase about thirty seconds each day after that. This enables you to progress without pain or injury. Your program depends on your goals. Goals might be weight loss, longevity, strength, muscle tone, flexibility, reducing cardiovascular risk factors, reducing depression and anxiety, rehabilitation from coronary heart disease, back pain, or sports performance.

CHAPTER 5

WHAT TO DO WHEN YOU FALL OFF THE WAGON

WHAT STAGE ARE YOU IN?

It might be that week when you have back-to-back out-of-town meetings followed by a deadline you can't miss. Or when the three year old gets an ear infection, the seven year old strep throat, and you have eight people coming for dinner on Friday.

Whatever the cause or excuse, there comes a time when you find yourself not exercising. It is then you should step back, reevaluate your motivation, and again figure out which stage of change you're in. Have you retrogressed to I Don't Want to Exercise? Have you only gone back as far as Thinking About It or Getting Ready?

Presumably before you fell off the wagon, you were in either the Starting or Keeping On stage. So just how far back have you fallen? Let's say that you've had a nasty cold. You've recovered, but you just haven't gotten back to exercising yet. If you're really just at the stage where you physically could begin again, you're still in Keeping On. The only thing to do then is that—keep on. The cold was a short detour. You've come back to the highway, so start exercising again.

What if you were really physically ready to start again two or three days ago, but you haven't gotten around to it? You're still in the stage of Keeping On and may just need a little boost to get you going again. You might visit your usual exercise haunt and see if that puts you in the mood.

If that's not enough to get you going, try positive self-statements. Say to yourself, "I enjoy exercising [or bicycling, or whatever it is you do]. It makes me feel better. It helps me [control my weight, or move more easily—you can fill in a reason or two]." Repeat this to yourself five times early in the morning, or whenever you think of it during the day, and just before bed. Don't get carried away and repeat the self-statements all day. Thirty times is plenty. Once you're back in the exercise habit, you can stop the self-statements.

STARTING

If this doesn't work, or if you have stayed away from exercise for a week or more without physical cause (injury, illness), you may have slid back to Starting.

The techniques to jump start you now are the same ones you used to move from Getting Ready to Starting and from Starting to Keeping On.

Bonnie had been doing very well on her program of using the stationary bike, but after she recovered from the flu, she just couldn't face it again. It seemed too boring. She needed something new. The six-hundred-dollar fee at the local health club seemed like a lot, but they had everything she wanted: a wide variety of aerobic equipment, weight machines, aero-

bic classes, a pool, and other things. She decided to take the plunge and paid the money. Unlike many people who pay and don't go, this commitment to act reinvigorated her exercise program.

Reinforcement management, helping relationships, and stimulus control can all be helpful too. Review these techniques in Chapter 2.

LEARN FROM PROBLEMS

Alan Marlatt's approach is quite helpful here. The first step toward resolving your problem is to realize you have one. Congratulate yourself for getting this far.

The next step is to tell yourself this is a normal part of the process and an opportunity for learning what to do this time and next. It's a chance to observe yourself, get a little more insight into your mind and how you approach the world.

To understand what you can learn from this episode, tell yourself it's not a catastrophe that you have not exercised for X number of days. The catastrophe would be considering it one and using that as an excuse to not exercise.

Retrace your steps. At exactly what point were you again capable of exercising but put it off? What day were you recovered enough from your cold/injury/busy period at work, or whatever interrupted you? What did you tell yourself that day about how you really couldn't exercise? How can you answer that objection today? Does that give you an answer that will be helpful the next time this problem comes back? You may feel silly talking to yourself, but you carry on internal dialogues all time—what should I wear? how should I apologize? what's the best approach for the presentation?

In this case, you're using the conversation with yourself to analyze what you're doing and why, coming to an understanding rather than floating along on a river of rationalization. What were the apparently irrelevant decisions that you made that led you to do other things in the time you set aside for exercise? What were the apparently irrelevant decisions you made the next day? The next day? Yesterday? Today?

The first three days might have been a busy period at the office. Then came preparing for a holiday at home and extra errands after work in the time you usually exercised. Then it was the weekend and visits to relatives and friends. Then came Monday and you were feeling out of shape and fat.

The most important thing for you at this point is to get back on track. It doesn't matter what happened last week. There's no changing the past—unless you're a former head of state writing your memoirs—it's the present that counts. You've got a modicum of control over that. You can say to yourself, "Okay self, the next thing I can do is to exercise today." You must not try to make up the lost days by pushing yourself until you're sore. Follow the Lazy Person's formula—take how many minutes it was you worked out the last time and subtract thirty seconds for each day over three you missed.

Then you can use the insights learned from examining the apparently irrelevant decisions from all those days you didn't exercise to help you get back on the wagon earlier next time and to goad yourself to exercise tomorrow.

By the time you're in the Keeping On stage, you'll actually feel exercise withdrawal when you stop for four days or more. Some depression strikes and you feel at loose ends. This improves when you start to exercise again.

GETTING HURT

As much as we'd like to tell you otherwise, you will have minor injuries. Other exercisers will talk about "working through the injury." You may have a brief minor discomfort that will disappear after a few minutes of exercise, but actual injuries are not "worked through." If you have an injury, either rest it until you can resume exercise or pursue exercise that does not use that body part.

Some injuries need to be seen by a physician and treated. There's nothing sissy about going to the doctor. Anytime you can't move a joint, you need to see a physician. With today's sports medicine approach, with medical consultation, you may be able to continue to exercise while protecting the injury and avoiding further damage.

You must learn to distinguish between discomfort and pain. Sharp pain or persistent dull pain is to be avoided. If there are sprained ligaments or irritated tendons, they often are painless long before they're fully healed. Caution and protection are required for at least six weeks after such injuries. On the other hand, some minor muscle discomfort is a normal part of beginning vigorous exercise.

Just don't use the injury as an excuse longer than it's valid.

CHAPTER 5 SUMMARY: When you fall off the wagon, first reassess your motivation. Most of the time you'll be in the Starting stage. Use strategies appropriate to that stage, or to the stage you're in, to get going again. Also use the principles of learning from problems. Don't beat yourself up for not exercising. This can lead to punishing yourself by not exercising even more. Use the problem as an opportunity to learn how it happened and how to avoid another similar problem the next time.

CHAPTER 6

RESISTANCE EXERCISE

Nope. This has nothing to do with the Scarlet Pimpernel or brave French underground fighters during World War II. Where muscles are concerned, resistance exercise means applying some impediment or obstruction as a counterforce to the muscles trying to contract. Muscles contract and generally shorten (they can also lengthen but more on that later) when they're used to move a joint.

If resistance is applied repeatedly for several weeks, the muscles will enlarge, and the resistance will be easier to overcome. This is strengthening. As your strength improves, so does the endurance of the muscles which is what allows us to perform repetitive motions for a long time. (Paddy Doyle can tell you about endurance—he holds the record for one-arm push-ups, 7,643 in one hour.)

Improved endurance could mean climbing stairs with less effort or shelling and eating a pound of peanuts without your arm getting tired, though that might not be such a great reason for boosting your stamina. Increased strength means increased muscle power which adds the factor of "time" to our discussion. Does it take two minutes to climb a flight of stairs or thirty seconds?

All right, so resistance exercise increases strength, endurance, and power. That sounds good. What next? What exactly is resistance exercise?

First you have to keep in mind that muscles move joints, and a joint is a moving part of the body composed of at least two bones. Place this book open on your lap or on a table. Hold the two sides with your right and left hands, your thumbs on the top. Where the page meets the crook of your hand is a joint.

You can manipulate the pages in a number of ways. Close the book from left to right, right to left, fold either page back so cover meets cover, swivel the book up or down. Think of your muscles as a set of springs stretching from one side of the book to the other, both on top and underneath.

Now the fun begins and we see how muscles work and what various types of resistive exercises we can perform. Contract the "springs" of your hands, that is shorten them, at the same time so that the book won't move. Even though there is no movement, your muscles are working and therefore strengthening. This is an **ISOMETRIC** exercise.

Another isometric exercise would be trying to open and close one side of the book as it's held by an immovable force. In other words, you're exerting force while seemingly accomplishing nothing. In fact, over time you'll get stronger from your futile efforts.

Instead of that immovable force, put something like a paperweight on the page. You can open and close the book but with difficulty. This is called an **ISOTONIC** resistance exercise. Strengthening is increased by using a heavier paperweight.

In isotonic resistance, movement occurs from the effort of the springs to shorten or close the book. In lifting the right side of the book with the paperweight, there is a concentric or shortening muscle contraction. When lowering that side to the table, as long as you don't let it drop, your muscles keep working to allow for a slow descent. The muscle is still contracting, but it's lengthening at the same time. This is called an eccentric contraction. Both types of isotonic resistance exercises are helpful in building strength and can easily be performed at home, work, or wherever.

ISOKINETIC is another type of resistance exercise. Here the important factor is not the weight of the object but how fast it's moving. Suppose there is a very powerful invisible motor opening and closing the book at a very precise speed. No matter what you do, you can't stop the book but you can still exert pressure in trying, thereby strengthening your muscles. You can control the effort of your muscles. You can just go along for the ride and let your hands move back and forth with the book, or you can attempt to stop the infernal motor with your muscles giving their all.

Another example of isokinetic exercise is to envision the powerful invisible motor not moving one side of the book but preventing the book from opening or closing in any faster than, say, ten seconds. So, try as you might with all your strength, ten seconds would always be required to open or close the book. You would provide your own resistance. If you tried to close the book in two seconds, you would have to make a tremendous effort and thus the muscle would strengthen.

While this type of exercise has many benefits and can probably match most exactly what our muscles are required to do in real life, very powerful invisible motors can't be found on every street corner or Sears home fitness department. Some gyms and physical therapists do have isokinetic exercise devices. But don't rush into using one without first receiving careful knowledgeable instruction.

PRECAUTIONS

The precautions we recommend for the Lazy Person are mostly plain common sense. You're out to feel better and look better, not to cripple yourself.

First off, if you feel there's any risk involved in your exercising—you have heart or breathing problems, joint or muscle difficulties, are taking regular medication, or suffer from or suspect you suffer from a disease—be sure to consult with your doctor before beginning a fitness program.

Also, avoid exercising if you're running a temperature. Ligaments are easily overstretched when you have a fever, which probably accounts for some of the muscle and joint aches and pains associated with one. And of course, if you have any pain while exercising, stop immediately.

One of the most basic precautions is to avoid the Valsalva's maneuver. The what? That's the effort to breathe out while keeping your windpipe shut. The grunt or yell that accompanies tremendous effort by weight lifters or martial arts enthusiasts is a method to ensure that their windpipe is open. So don't hold your breath while performing isometric or heavy resistance exercise. Holding your breath builds up pressure in your chest area and abdomen and can have harmful side effects on your heart and circulation. The easiest way to avoid a Valsalva's maneuver is to *COUNT OUT LOUD* while you perform your resistive exercise. You may not even realize that you're holding your breath, though anyone watching you would see your face flush and darken. Talk or count and you'll breathe.

Another no-no is overfatiguing yourself during exercise. This is when being a Lazy Person is very useful. Don't overdo it. That's *OVER*do it. Your muscles are going to slow down some and weaken over the course of an exercise session. That's normal, and even the Lazy Person has to live with that. What isn't normal is when you demand too much of a fatigued muscle. That's when injuries occur. And it doesn't matter if you're doing isometric or static exercise. You don't need to be a rocket scientist or a physical therapist to know when your muscle has had enough. You're going to get that unpleasant feeling of your body protesting "enough, already, enough," and sometimes there's even pain and spasm.

Overall or general body fatigue is another precaution to consider. This comes after a prolonged activity such as jogging or walking. Even a low-intensity workout if done for a long time can cause fatigue and thus make you vulnerable to injury. Fatigue can also occur if there is an underlying heart or breathing problem or many other conditions. Besides getting your doctor's okay if you have any such conditions, it would probably be wise to consult a physical or occupational therapist before exercising.

Okay, so what should you do if you're in the middle of your exercise routine, and suddenly, you're body-slammed with exhaustion? Easy. Slow down, then stop.

Generally a cool-down period of very light or easy exercise allows for faster recovery than simply stopping outright. Muscles require a rest to replenish their energy. Some of the energy stores require a day or two to rebuild to preexercise levels. Also waste products build up in the muscle during exercise (lactic acid). At least one hour is required for the body to cleanse the muscle after exercise. By all means avoid the "No pain, no gain," "No squeal, no heal" school of thought. Overdoing it can cause temporary or even a permanent reduction in strength.

Avoid excessive muscle soreness. After a strenuous exercise bout, there is an increase of lactic acid and a decrease in the usual amount of oxygen. This should subside quickly. More prolonged soreness can last for a few days after a really strenuous workout but gradually diminishes. This extended soreness probably results from those small tears in the muscle, which take time to heal. A proper warm-up and cool-down and a gradual increase in resistance can reduce the soreness. Every fall with leaf raking and every winter with snow shoveling, people visit us with complaints of sore backs, legs, and arms. Even the most sedentary Lazy Person springs into frenzied action at the sight of snow or piling leaves. Rosa, a sixty-seven-year-old woman who had fallen and fractured a bone in her back a month previously, was in Dave's office complaining of a sore back after chipping ice from her driveway for two hours. The look in her eyes suggested that his advice to avoid shoveling would be forgotten as soon as the next flake hit the pavement.

CHAPTER 6 SUMMARY: Isotonic exercises are performed moving against resistance, such as raising and lowering a weight-machine handle or barbell at your own pace. Isometric exercises are performed without moving, pushing or pulling against a stationary object. Isokinetic exercises are performed pushing or pulling against an object that moves at a set rate of speed. Isokinetic exercises require highly specialized equipment. Always avoid holding your breath (Valsalva's maneuver) when exercising. Avoid pain and soreness.

CHAPTER 7

ISOMETRICS

"Let's see that muscle!" From the time we're small, it's realized we can *make* a muscle. Popeye made a career of frightening Bluto with his muscle making and fortifying his popping biceps with cans of spinach.

Tensing a muscle without any movement of your body is called isometrics. That's how we *make* a muscle. Isometrics are the easiest and simplest ways to start exercising. Since there's no movement, you can do isometric exercises any-place with little or no equipment. The muscle that you select contracts or tightens but does not change length, thus there is no movement of the joint or the bones to which the muscle is attached.

Isometric exercise can be performed against resistance or by simply *setting* the muscle. Of course, you have to be careful about what you do and where you do it. One of Dave's patients engaged in some isometric muscle activity much to his detriment. This sixty-five-year-old gentleman had a flat tire one evening and rather than wait for AAA to show up, decided to change it himself. The only problem was that the lug nuts were rusted and not about to move. The determined gentleman tugged and pulled with his wrench to no avail.

Finally he positioned himself so that he could use his strong thigh muscles in his battle to free the nuts. He maintained his elbow and biceps muscle in a fixed position while holding the lug wrench. With a mighty heave, he straightened his knees. Unfortunately it was his biceps muscles and not the rusted nuts that gave way.

Generally, however, isometrics are safe and easy. Dave's patient made the mistake of applying the force of his strong leg muscles and expecting his weaker biceps muscles to bear the burden. If he had used only his biceps muscles in his attempt to loosen the nut, there would have been no tear. Of course, the nut wouldn't have budged either, but it would have taken less time for him to wait for AAA than it took his body to repair itself. So learn from the gentleman's misfortune. With isometrics, the muscle should be working on its own without the help of other parts of the body in an attempt to create greater forces.

These exercises are an easy way to increase strength. Great amounts of torque or force can be developed by using this method. In fact, you can apply more force this way than when the muscle is moving and shortening (a concentric muscle contraction). While isometrics will dramatically increase the strength of the muscle, it will not increase your endurance as much as exercises where you move. (Isometrics or "dynamic tension" techniques were popularized a few decades ago by Charles "Sand in the Face" Atlas. While many of the associated claims of besting bullies and developing a magnetic personality were overblown, the exercise principle was real.)

Before beginning a program of isometrics, you should keep in mind—better still, carve them on your brain—several important points.

1. AVOID PAIN! No exercise should cause joint or muscle pain. A sense of effort or mild discomfort that doesn't last long is okay, but *no pain*. This is especially true for you, the Lazy Person, who looks for any and every excuse to stop exercising.

2. NEVER HOLD YOUR BREATH. Remember this is especially true while performing isometric and heavy resistance exercise. The easiest way to avoid a Valsalva's blue-in-the-face maneuver is to *COUNT OUT LOUD* while exercising. That doesn't mean you have to scream so that everyone within four city blocks is dialling 911. But do make your counting audible. This forces you to breathe.

3. TIGHTEN THE MUSCLE SLOWLY WHILE YOU COUNT OUT LOUD TO FIVE. Make each count a second, for example, say, "One thousand one, one thousand two..." to approximate one second per count. When you begin this type of muscle strengthening, begin slowly and build your effort to a peak. Think of a car starting from a stoplight. You don't reach fifty-five miles per hour immediately (not even dragsters do). It takes a few seconds, hence the zero to sixty statistic that's bandied about. The same is the case for your muscle as you count out loud to five. By the time you reach the number four, you should be exerting your optimum force.

It's important to hold the effort because the muscle then has time to build up tension, and you get some of the changes necessary to occur within the muscle to improve strength.

4. AIM FOR A 75% EFFORT. Strengthening will occur in isometrics using 75 percent of your maximum force. Granted it's difficult to determine exactly what the maximum force of your particular muscle is because several factors are involved. The muscle you're targeting is the most important factor. The muscles used to spread your fingers apart versus those used to straighten a bent knee have vastly different force capacities. Your maximum effort, however, in pushing with these muscles is the *same.* Your goal is to push as hard as you can, no matter which muscle you are exercising, but stop just short of that all-out effort.

5. DO 5 REPETITIONS. Muscles need to be stressed in order to strengthen. The muscles can then develop greater levels of tension and force. An adequate number of repetitions to achieve the strengthening effect is five. So when you perform the isometrics, tighten the muscle five times, each to the count of five.

6. CHANGE POSITIONS. Isometric strengthening tends to build strength mainly in the position that you exercise. To build up the whole muscle, you have to change the joint position. Your elbow can be straight with your palm down (reaching for some popcorn) or the elbow can be bent with the palm up (putting same in your mouth). Isometric exercises in the various positions of your palm and your elbow on the way from the bowl to your mouth will strengthen many muscles in your arm. It's also important to remember that muscles have less strength when the joint they control is at the end of its motion. So in the popcorn example, the elbow muscles are less strong with the elbow fully straightened or fully bent.

7. GET THE ONE YOU WANT. When performing isometric exercises, it's important to make sure you strengthen the muscle you've targeted. In general this means you should see and feel the muscle work. Try and push or pull against some unmovable force with a part of your body that only involves one joint. For example, if you're trying to strengthen your biceps (Popeye) arm muscle, by bending your elbow, then you should be stopping your wrist from moving, not your fingers. If you were pushing or pulling with your fingers and trying to bend the elbow, the wrist, finger, and elbow muscles would all be working. If you divide your effort this way, the stronger biceps muscle wouldn't get a maximum workout, and the fingers would be overworked.

8. FLIP-FLOP. Don't forget that most muscles have a counterpart that performs the opposite activity. In the case of popcorn eating, you would be using opposing muscles depending on which direction you were headed. Reaching for the bowl would use the triceps (back of the elbow) and stuffing a few kernels in your mouth would employ the biceps (front of the elbow). Do isometrics that stop motion in both directions when doing your strengthening. Similar opposites exist for all the muscles that you might be working on.

77

9. ANYTIME-ANYPLACE. The beauty of isometric exercises is that you can perform them anytime and anyplace. Home, the office, or school are all easily turned into a strength-building gym for your instant workout. Once you localize what you want to strengthen, the possibilities are endless for designing your own methods of isometric exercise. They can be done in such a way that no one will even realize that you're exercising, except for the counting out loud, which you can replace with conversation. Even on the phone or in a meeting, your strengthening can proceed. Daily workouts, which take little if any time, will quickly build your muscles. Do a "Tale of the Tape" (stretch a tape measure around the biggest part of your muscle) to compare your muscle girth before and after your exercising if you aren't yet convinced.

10. HEAD TO TOE. Your objective will be to strengthen and tone muscles from head to toe. We will shortly go over a few of the many different muscles you can strengthen and some of the various positions you can use. Remember, just about any muscle can be strengthened this way, and there are a host of positions that can be tailored to fit your particular situation.

11. HOW OFTEN. There are several theories on how often you should exercise isometrically. **Some have advocated just one maximal effort held for five seconds, once a day, five days a week.**** A less extreme approach would be to perform five maximal efforts, held for five seconds, once a day, five days a week. The five-repetition approach would allow

***A Lazy Person's Guide to Fitness* Top Choice

you to use the muscle at slightly different angles, and therefore strengthen more of the muscle.

REMEMBER—STOP IF YOU HAVE ANY PAIN AND CONSULT A PROFESSIONAL.

Okay, enough of definitions, admonitions, and generalized counsel. It's Show Time, time for real live isometric exercises for the Lazy Person, body part by body part.

HEAD

MUSCLES: All the muscles that support your head (fifteen pounds) and neck. These are muscles that were targeted for strengthening by the postural school of balancing a book on you head while walking.

(What person can't remember their mother admonishing them to sit up or stand straight? If you want to know if you are, have someone look at you from the side and see if your ear is lined up straight on top of the tip of your shoulder. It should be if your head is straight.)

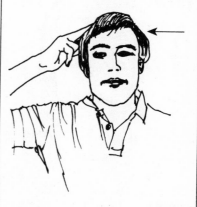

FIGURE 3

METHOD: Place 2 fingers on the front of your forehead and push forward. DO NOT ALLOW YOUR HEAD TO MOVE! Only 2 fingers are needed to provide resistance to the neck muscles. Do your 5 repetitions, counting out loud to 5 each time. Now move your fingers to the back, left, and then right side of you head and repeat. (See figure 3.) This is great for the office. Your coworkers will think you're thinking.

RESULTS: Neck muscles that will support your head in maintaining good posture during the day's activities. Especially important for those at a desk for long periods at the office or school.

FACE

MUSCLES: All the muscles that mold your face into the whole gamut of human emotions and expressions. Joy, sorrow, laughter, tears, and wonder are expressed by a combination of facial muscles. Disregard the age-old adage of "how would you like your face to freeze like that?"

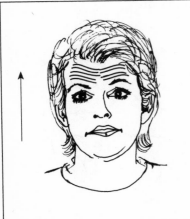

FIGURE 4

METHOD: Pick an expression—frowning (eyebrows down), wrinkling your forehead (eyebrows up), wrinkling your nose, pulling your lips back to show your teeth, pulling down your lower lip and feeling all the muscles of your chin and neck work, or any other facial movement that you can manage. Make the face and hold it for 5 seconds, 5 times. (See figure 4.)

RESULTS: Firms facial muscles, eases tension built up from maintaining static positions for long periods. Provides a more varied expression and interaction with those around you. A window to the soul.

SHOULDERS

MUSCLES: The muscles that operate the shoulder "girdle." These muscles operate the shoulder blades and your arms.

The shoulder is called the "great" joint because of its ability to move in so many different ways. Its chief function is to enable you to place your hand in the numerous and nearly unlimited positions required to perform your daily activities. (You can scratch the middle of your back, reach up and pat the top of your head, or delicately toss a token into a toll basket from a moving car.) The ball of the shoulder is held in the shallow shoulder socket mainly by muscles and ligaments. Keeping the muscles strong prevents injuries and allows for fun and top performance during most recreational activities, especially racquet sports and golfing. Strong shoulder muscles also help in good posture. "Pull those shoulders back" is another childhood instruction that we all too quickly forget. And last but not least, they're helpful in reaching for the remote control so that you can indulge in your favorite sport—channel surfing.

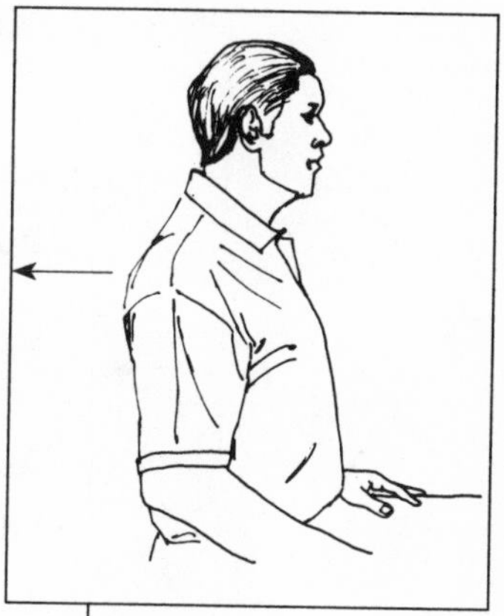

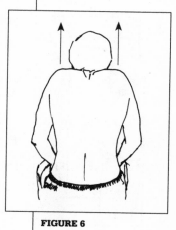

FIGURE 5

METHOD: The blades

1. Standing or sitting, pull your shoulder blades together, or your shoulders back, however you wish to think of it. Count out loud to—you guessed it—5, 5 times. (See figure 5.)

2. Shrug or lift your shoulders up toward your ears and hold. Count out loud to 5, 5 times. (See figure 6.)

3. Pull your shoulders forward, like you're trying to round your back, and hold. Count out loud to 5, 5 times. (See figure 7.)

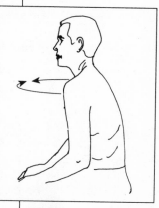

FIGURE 6

FIGURE 7

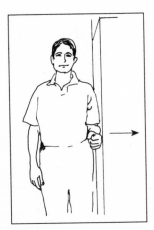

FIGURE 8

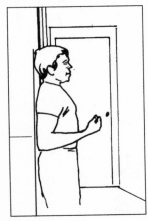

FIGURE 9

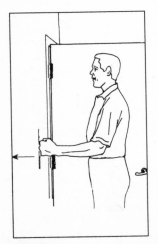

FIGURE 10

METHOD: The shoulders

There are 5 basic movements performed with your elbow at your side and bent at 90 degrees. Make believe you're holding your hand out for another snack. You can do these either sitting or standing.

1. With your elbow at your side, push your arm out against a wall or the arm of your chair. Place your arm inside the arm of the chair when pushing out. (This technique is helpful when trying to enter a crowded subway car or exit a football stadium.) Try and move your elbow out away from your side but make the wall or chair prevent you from doing so. Count out loud to 5, 5 times. (See figure 8.)

2. Keep your elbow bent with your hand in front of you, and push your elbow back into the wall or chair and hold. (Useful muscles to have for the backward "don't touch me" move in a crowded elevator.) Count out loud to 5, 5 times. (See figure 9.)

3. Hold your wrist with your other hand, push forward against your desk or grab a doorframe and push forward. Don't let your arm move. You will feel the muscles in the front of your shoulder working and strengthening. (Ideal muscles to use when attempting to push open an outside door on a windy day in Chicago along Lake Michigan.) Count out loud to 5, 5 times. (See figure 10.)

4. With your elbow at 90 degrees at your side just as you did above, block your wrist with your other hand, the corner of your desk, or a doorjamb. Try hard to put your hand on your stomach without moving the arm. (This group of muscles will allow you to collect any size pile of poker chips with ease or drag a distant heavy plate of food nearer to your

plate.) You'll feel your front shoulder and chest muscles working. Count out loud to 5, 5 times. (See figure 11.)

5. And the last for the shoulder. Try and do just the opposite of number 4 above. Make the effort as if you were trying to move your hand out from your body away from your stomach. Don't let the arm move! Keep the elbow at your side. Count out loud to 5, 5 times. (See figure 12.)

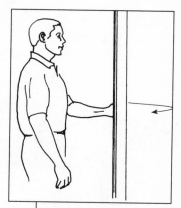

FIGURE 11

RESULTS: The above exercises strengthen the muscles around the shoulder without putting undo strain on this delicate joint. Strong shoulder muscles help with posture, improve sports activities that involve throwing or using a racquet, and improves the fit of your Armani sport jacket.

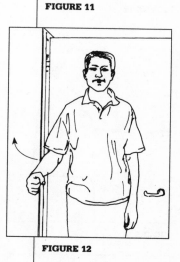

FIGURE 12

ARMS

MUSCLES: Mainly the muscles that bend and straighten the elbow. Very useful for lifting objects and pushing yourself up out of your Naugahyde lounge chair (unless, of course, you have an automatic-seat chair lift).

METHOD:

1. Grab the top of your wrist, palm up, with the other hand, or place your wrist under your desk and try to bend your elbow. Your hand should be trying to move up toward your shoulder. Don't let it! Count out loud to 5, 5 times. (See figure 13.)

2. Hold the back of your wrist still palm up or place it on top of a table, a desk, or your knee if sitting, and try to

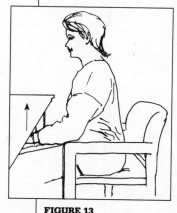

FIGURE 13

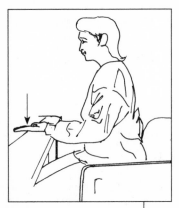

FIGURE 14

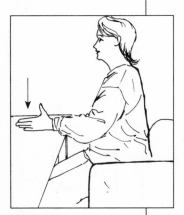

FIGURE 15

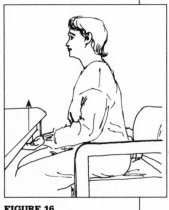

FIGURE 16

straighten your elbow. Don't let it move! Count out loud to 5, 5 times. (See figure 14.)

3. If you're adventuresome, use the thumb up in No. 1 and 2 instead of the wrist. Don't move and count out loud to 5, 5 times. (See figure 15.)

RESULTS: Builds up your Popeye biceps on the front of the arm and the triceps on the back. These are frequently used as benchmark muscles to gauge overall condition.

HANDS

MUSCLES: The many muscles lying between the elbow and the wrist that control the wrists and fingers. These are capable of great strength and endurance as well as extremely delicate movements such as cracking Macadamia nuts and then carefully extracting the contents. These muscles are our chief means of interacting with our environment and those around us. Improper use or weakness of this group can cause numerous ailments ranging from tennis or golf elbows and carpal tunnel syndrome—the check-out grocery clerk and computer terminal operator's nemesis—to more exotic maladies such as gamekeeper's thumb (caused by lugging around a bunch of dead birds attached to a rope hanging down your back).

METHOD:

1. Place one hand on the palm of the other or put your palm face up under a desk or table. Keep your wrist straight

and use your palm, not your fingers. Then, try and bend your wrist up toward your head. Count out loud to 5, 5 times. Slowly increase your effort over the 5 counts. (See figure 16.)

2. Modify the above exercise by placing the resistance on the back of your hand instead of the palm. Try to bend your wrist backwards. Don't let the wrist move, but you would be heading toward the wrist position a waiter has when carrying a tray over his shoulder. Do the regular count, to 5, 5 times. (See figure 17.)

3. Various finger isometric exercises:

Place the fingers of one hand straight and together. Press the outside of your straight pinkie and index finger with your other hand. (An excellent group of muscles to strengthen for you magicians who open their hands wide to show the coin has disappeared.) Try to separate your straight fingers without actually accomplishing it to the count of 5. Repeat 5 times. (See figure 18.)

Interlock your fingers (not on the knuckles) and squeeze the fingers together. This allows you to exercise both hands at once. (See figure 19.)

You can design other finger strengthening exercises for yourself. Remember there should be no movement despite the effort and above all NO PAIN!!!

RESULTS: Strong forearms, wrists, and fingers. Essential for both endurance and fine work. You don't want to poop out in the third quarter of a Cowboys-Eagles game while you're separating the nuts from that other stuff in Trail

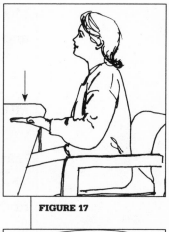

FIGURE 17

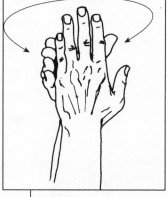

FIGURE 18

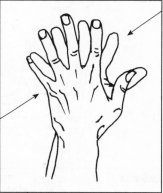

FIGURE 19

Mix. Stronger hands will get you through an entire pound and may also save you from tennis and golf elbow.

BACK

MUSCLES: The two main opposing muscle groups that control the back are the long strong muscles along your spine that hold you erect and the stomach or abdominal muscles. The abdominals act to support the internal organs and the front of your spine. Both are very important for good posture and avoiding back pain. Some studies have shown that nearly 80 percent of working men and women will suffer back pain at some point in their adult lives. The pain will be enough to keep them out of work. **If you have lower back problems, don't do these exercises until you've consulted your physician or physical therapist.**

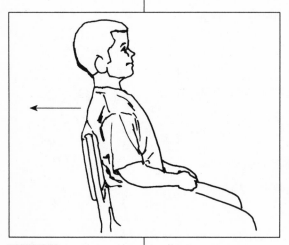

FIGURE 20

METHOD:

1. Sitting in your chair or standing against a wall, try and straighten your back by pushing into the chair or wall. Remember to breathe when you are doing this 5 times for a count of 5. This exercise will strengthen your back extensor muscles. Besides being strong, they need to have the endurance to allow you to sit erect during the day. (See figure 20.)

2. Another way to strengthen back muscles is to lie on your stomach with your arms at your side and lift your shoulders and head up from the bed and hold. (This motion would

be the one to use at the beach to check for a rising tide, that ubiquitous sand-kicking bully, or Claudia Schiffer sauntering by.) Keep your neck straight, don't bend your head back. You only have to raise up an inch or two to get the desired effect. Count out loud to 5, 5 times. (See figure 21.)

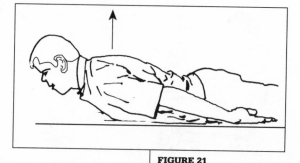

FIGURE 21

3. When sitting or standing, pull your stomach in, hold, and do the count. You'll be able to feel your stomach muscles working. (This is generally only done when trying on a pair of old jeans that have mysteriously shrunk several sizes.) Keep your lower back straight and slightly arched during these stomach exercises. (See figure 22.)

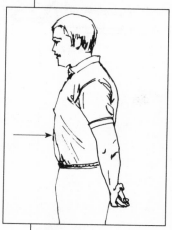

FIGURE 22

4. Lying on your back with your knees bent and feet on the bed or floor (don't hook your feet under anything), cross your arms on your chest and lift your head and shoulders just slightly up from the bed. (This is popularly called doing "crunches.") Hold this position while you count out loud to 5, 5 times. (See figure 23.)

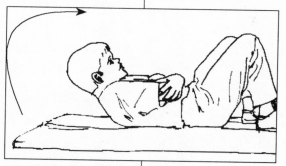

FIGURE 23

RESULTS: These exercises help maintain good posture which is essential for proper back care. For those of you who sit for long periods during the day, keeping your lower back slightly arched and supported will help immensely. Firm abdominal muscles give support for the lower back and have a firm flat appearance.

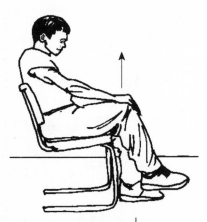

HIPS

MUSCLES: All of the muscles that surround the hip joint. Some are very powerful and have great endurance. They're also some of the largest in the body, for example, the gluteus maximus, otherwise known as buttocks, buns, or tush. Generally in need of firming for all the lazy exercisers out there.

METHOD: Sitting

1. Hold your knee with one or both of your hands and attempt to lift your foot off the floor. (Remember, this is an isometric exercise. Don't let your knee actually move.) Make sure you're sitting with good posture. You'll feel the muscle work in the front of your hip. Count out loud to 5, 5 times. (See figure 24.)

2. Place your knee or the side of your leg against something firm, like your desk, a table, or the side of your chair. Push out as if trying to spread your knees apart. Don't let your leg move. Make sure the table is sturdy, these muscles are quite strong and are on the side of your hip. Count out loud to 5, 5 times. (See figure 25.)

3. Place a book or rolled-up towel between your knees and squeeze together. This strengthens the inner thigh muscles. Count out loud to 5, 5 times. (See figure 26.)

METHOD: Standing

1. Stand in a doorway (nonchalantly, if you don't want the entire accounting department to know you're exer-

cising) with the side of one leg against the jamb. Push your leg straight out to the side. Your toes should be pointed forward but your effort to move will be sideways. Count out loud to 5, 5 times. (See figure 27.)

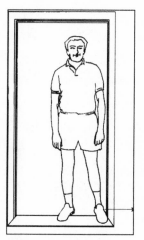

FIGURE 27

2. Keep standing in the doorway, but now place the back of one leg against the doorframe and push backwards. You should feel your buttock muscles working. Count out loud to 5, 5 times. (See figure 28.)

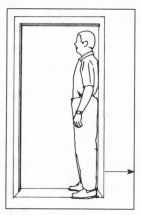

FIGURE 28

3. Turn again so that the front of one leg is facing and touching the doorframe. Push that leg forward. This exercises the front hip muscles. Count out loud to 5, 5 times. (See figure 29.)

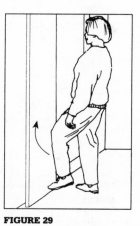

FIGURE 29

4. And last, stand in the doorway close to and facing the doorframe. Hold on if you like. Move one leg forward so that the inside of your thigh is against the wall. It will be like you're going to cross one leg over the other, but the wall stops you. (Now might be the time to confess to accounting that you're exercising, otherwise there may be some strange conjecturing about you at coffee break.) Try and pull your leg in toward the other leg. You'll feel your inside thigh muscles work. Count out loud to 5, 5 times. (See figure 30.)

RESULTS: This series of exercises performed either sitting or standing strengthen many of the most important hip muscles. You will have an easier time walking, climb steps better, and while these exercises may not provide *Buns of Steel,* your thighs and hips will be more shapely.

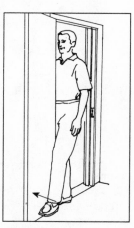

FIGURE 30

KNEES

MUSCLES: The "quads," or quadriceps, are the four muscles that make up the very powerful group on the front of your thigh. The opposing group, the "hams," or hamstrings, are the three almost-as-powerful muscles that are on the back of the thigh. These muscles waste away, or atrophy, very quickly, so it's important for the Lazy Person to use them for more than walking from the front door to the car or from the kitchen to the TV. The nice thing about these groups of muscles is that they build up and strengthen quite quickly and easily. "Hamstringing" as a synonym for hampering or impeding one's activities arises from the ancient art of cutting the hamstring tendons of captured prisoners to guard them more easily. When the hamstrings are unattached, it becomes very difficult to walk quickly, and running away becomes all but impossible.

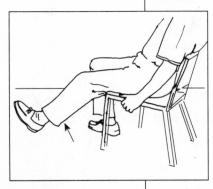

FIGURE 31

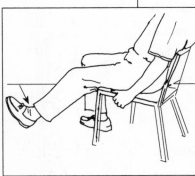

FIGURE 32

METHOD: Sitting

QUADRICEPS—Stretch out your leg with your heel on the floor and your knee almost straight. Try to straighten your knee without letting it move. You'll feel the powerful front thigh muscles tighten. Count out loud to 5, 5 times. (See figure 31.)

HAMSTRINGS—Place your heel on the floor about one foot in front of your chair. Push your heel into the floor. You'll feel the muscles on the back of the thigh tighten. Count out loud to 5, 5 times. (See figure 32.)

QUADS AND HAMS—Sit with your legs crossed at the ankles. Try and straighten out the back leg while preventing any movement with the front leg. This technique will strengthen the quadriceps of the back leg and the hamstrings of the front leg at the same time. Then reverse the crossed ankles. Count out loud to 5, 5 times. (See figure 33.)

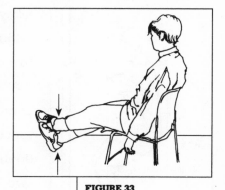

FIGURE 33

LYING ON YOUR BACK—Bend one knee and place your foot flat on the bed or floor. Straighten the other leg with the knee slightly bent and the heel on the bed. Then push the back of your knee down into the bed or floor but DON'T LET IT MOVE. You will feel both the hamstrings and the quadriceps contract. Count out loud to 5, 5 times. (See figure 34.)

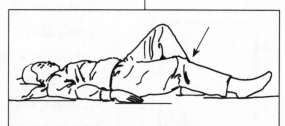

FIGURE 34

LYING ON YOUR STOMACH—Bend both knees slightly, bringing them about twelve inches off the bed or floor. Cross your ankles and then try straightening the top leg. Use the bottom leg to prevent any movement. This, again, will strengthen the quads of the top leg and the hams of the bottom. Count out loud to 5, 5 times. (See figure 35.)

METHOD: Standing

QUADRICEPS—Hold onto something, like a doorframe, for balance, with your feet about a two feet apart. Keep your lower back straight, as if you were going to sit in a chair. Then, bend your knees slightly. Keep your heels on the ground, and don't

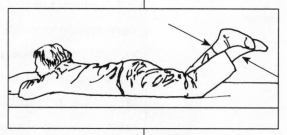

FIGURE 35

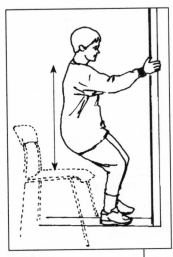

FIGURE 36

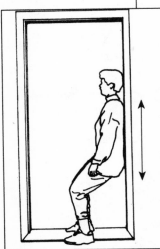

FIGURE 37

let your knees touch the doorframe. This prevents undue strain on you kneecaps. Hold it for the five and five count. (See figure 36.)

A VARIATION—Stand with your back to the wall and your feet apart and away from the wall. Slide your bottom down the wall toward a sitting position. Don't slide down as far as if you were in a chair, however. (These two exercises are commonly called "squats.") Count out loud to 5, straighten up a bit, and repeat 5 times. (See figure 37.)

RESULTS: These exercises are intended to provide strong thigh muscles. They will build up quite quickly, and in a few weeks, you'll see a difference in the shape of your thigh. Climbing steps will be easier with stronger knee muscles. Strong quadriceps and hamstrings are also thought to provide valuable protection to the easily injured knee joint.

ANKLES

MUSCLES: Let's start with the huge calf muscles, which are the ones that lift you up on your toes. They're very strong considering that they're lifting your entire body weight when you're on your toes. The calf muscles are attached to the heel bone by the Achilles tendon, of mythical fame as a vulnerable area of the body. This tendon was severed as a punishment for captured soldiers in ancient times because when severed, you lose that "bounce" in your step, to put it mildly, and in fact cannot run or even walk very well.

The next important ankle group is the shin muscles. These lift up your foot and toe when walking. They prevent your toe and foot from dragging.

The other main ankle muscles are those that turn your foot in and out. A "pigeon-toed" position is achieved by using the invertors or turning-in muscles. The evertors would be used to toe out, as seen in the exaggerated form of some ballet positions with toes pointing east and west.

METHOD: Standing

THE CALVES—The easiest way to isometrically exercise the very strong calf muscles is to go up on your toes and stay there. You'll be supporting your entire body weight. Once you're comfortable doing that, lift one of your feet slightly off the floor. A friend of ours, John, has perfected this exercise and does it while putting on his pants every morning. He stands and balances on one foot while sliding his leg into the trousers and goes up on his toes to really strengthen his calf muscles. Count out loud to 5, 5 times. (See figure 38.)

THE SHIN—Lift your foot and toes so that you're supported on your heels alone. Hold on to something sturdy for balance, if necessary. Gradually, lift your feet with greater and greater effort. (An excellent technique for walking through puddles.) Your can do this with one foot at a time or with both at once. Count out loud to 5, 5 times. (See figure 39.)

IN AND OUT—Stand sideways next to a wall or, better yet, in a doorway facing the doorframe with the outside of

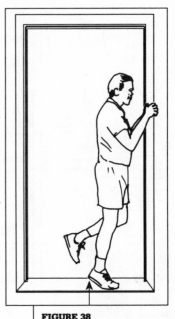

FIGURE 38

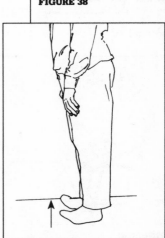

FIGURE 39

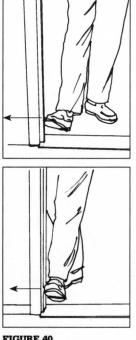

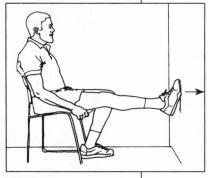

FIGURE 40

your foot firmly against the wall or frame. Push so that your foot is trying to move away from the other foot. You'll be trying to spread your legs apart, but the doorframe will stop you. Count out loud to 5, 5 times. This strengthens the turning-out muscles. Then position your foot (easier done against a doorframe) so that you're trying to turn your foot in toward the other foot. Don't let it move and then count out loud to 5, 5 times. (See figure 40.)

METHOD: Sitting

THE CALVES—If you can find a sturdy, substantial chair to sit in or can sit with your back against a wall, stretch your leg out so that your foot is against something unmovable (and unbreakable). Then push down with your foot as if you're stepping on the gas pedal. Push gradually harder and harder to strengthen the calf muscles. Count out loud to 5, 5 times. (See figure 41.)

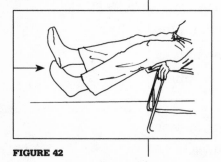

FIGURE 41

FIGURE 42

THE SHIN—Place the heel of one foot on the instep of the foot on the floor. Try and lift the toes and foot of the one underneath. Keep the bottom foot from moving with pressure from the top foot. Then reverse feet. Count out loud to 5, 5 times. (See figure 42.)

IN AND OUT—Place your feet together, toes pointing forward, and try pushing them together. Keep your knee slightly apart when doing this and make sure you only use your foot and ankle muscles. This covers the turning-in muscles. Then you can place the outside of your foot against a table leg or desk wall and try to turn your foot out away from the other one. As a slight variation, working both feet at once, cross your legs at the ankle so that the outside of your feet are touching and then push them together. Count out loud to 5, 5 times. (See figure 43.)

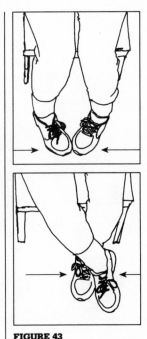

RESULTS: Strong ankle muscles help prevent strains and sprains when you suddenly twist your foot on an uneven sidewalk or plummet into a camouflaged pothole. Strong calf muscles produce a spring in your step and ease stair climbing if you're so inclined. Use of these muscles is also very helpful in improving circulation in the lower leg. And, of course, many people find a muscular or well-defined calf a thing of beauty or at least of admiration.

FIGURE 43

CHAPTER 7 SUMMARY: Isometrics increase strength dramatically, but not endurance. To perform isometrics, avoid pain, never hold your breath, tighten slowly while you count out loud to five, aim for a 75 percent effort. Do five repetitions, change positions, get the muscle you want. Flip-flop the opposing muscles, do them anytime and anyplace, work muscles from head to toe, and do them one to five times a day, up to five days a week.

CHAPTER 8

THE BASICS OF MOVEMENT EXERCISE

Now we have to consider some of the many hotly debated topics on the best ways to exercise. The various options are merely posed for your consideration. We'll combine all of the various theories and have them tailored to meet the Lazy Person's route to fitness and strength. Most of the basics will concern isotonic resistance (weight lifting) exercise or isokinetic exercise (velocity training).

The theories on how best to exercise answer the following questions:

How heavy a load do you lift?

How fast do you lift it?

How many repetitions of the effort do you perform?

How many times in one session do you perform the repetitions?

Should you change the amount of resistance when moving?

How often should you exercise each week?

How many weeks will it take to increase your strength?

HOW HEAVY A LOAD DO YOU LIFT? Even the laziest Lazy Person does *some* lifting. You pick up the newspaper from your driveway. You lift the plates out of the dishwasher. Why, you might even hoist a bag of groceries from the check-out counter into your basket. Unfortunately, none of that does much in the way of strengthening to your arm muscles. You're going to have to overwork that muscle—at least a little—if you want it stronger. That is, it must be difficult for the muscle to perform the task.

Before you panic, Lazy Person, no one is asking you to start lifting the equivalent of a Cadillac on your first day. You need to figure out how much weight is required to overload your muscles—and not those of the guy next to you who has arms bigger than your torso. It's not easy to determine exactly where that overload point is, but the rule of thumb is it's however much you can lift ten times without feeling you need a paramedic. Remember, this isn't supposed to hurt you. You know when your muscles are politely asking to be excused. That's when you've reached your maximal load. If you can only lift five pounds eight times, then lower the weight to four pounds so you can perform the ten repetitions.

Most of the time you'll be exercising submaximally and will gradually increase the amount of the resistance or weight. We're talking about a few pounds every week or so. This scenario is mainly designed to increase strength rather than endurance, but there is no definite way that is most effective for progressing your lifting.

There's no need to run out and buy a four-hundred-piece weight set that would take a forklift to get out of your car. You can make your own weights. Gather up all those pennies that are lying around in desk drawers, pockets, and under couch cushions, and put them in those nice paper rolls the banks give you. Three rolls of pennies (fifty pennies per roll) equal one pound. Tape rolls together, and you have a nice, compact, easily adjustable source of weights. A couple of rolls could be added each week if you wanted to increase the work the muscle is performing.

If penny weights aren't to your liking, sporting goods stores sell adjustable weight cuffs that can be attached to your arm or leg and fastened with a buckle or Velcro. These cuffs have several pockets into which you slip little one-pound ingots. That way you can build up the weight at your own pace and not have to purchase individual weights.

You can also fashion your own cuff with the penny-roll method. Just attach the rolls of pennies with strong tape to the outside of an old belt (it should look somewhat like a western holster with bullets) and wrap the belt onto your arm or leg. Make sure that the rolls of pennies are secure.

If you're using strong rubber bands for resistance, fold them in half to increase the difficulty of the exercise, or find stronger rubber bands.

Now you're ready to go. Right. But questions remain, like—

HOW MANY REPETITIONS OF THE EFFORT DO YOU PERFORM? There have been numerous studies conducted in search of the ideal number of repetitions for increasing strength. Most exercise protocols use ten repetitions, some advocate six, and others go up to fifteen. The number of repetitions can also be used to figure out what is necessary to overload the muscle to build strength and/or endurance.

It's probably best to combine the amount of resistance with the number of repetitions to find out what is best for you. Generally speaking, if you want to increase endurance, a high number of repetitions will be required. That means you'll have to lower the amount of weight that you're lifting. If strength is the primary goal, then fewer repetitions and increased weight is the way to go. The Lazy Person should figure on lots of repetitions while keeping the weight or resistance fairly low and constant.

HOW MANY TIMES (SETS) IN A SESSION TO PERFORM THE REPETITIONS? The number of times you perform your chosen repetitions in one exercise session are called "sets." For example, you could perform two sets of ten repetitions each. This would mean a total of twenty repetitions but broken up so that you do ten, rest, and then do the second ten. It's been shown that muscles can improve in strength and endurance with as few as one set of one maximum repetition (as mentioned in the isometric section.) Others feel that several sets of varying repetitions are required to increase muscle performance. This could be three sets of ten repetitions or two sets of twelve.

As a Lazy Person, you'll be somewhere in the middle. With the isometric exercises, you did five reps of five seconds—how could you forget "count out loud to five, five times"? For resistance exercises, you'll again do five and five—five sets of five repetitions. You should begin, of course, with only one set and build up slowly over several weeks to the five sets of five repetitions. Once you're at the twenty-five combined repetitions, you can increase the weight if you wish.

HOW OFTEN SHOULD YOU DO ISOTONIC EXERCISE EACH WEEK? At least in this area there is some general consensus of opinion. Our experience is that every other day is the best routine to follow. This will provide three or four days a week of strengthening exercise. This frequency allows for rest after the session and is essential if you're exercising at an overload or maximum level. The muscle needs time to recover from its workout. A different approach would include changing which area of your body you exercise from day to day. For example, arms one day, legs the next, and stomach/back the third.

HOW MANY WEEKS WILL IT TAKE TO INCREASE YOUR STRENGTH? This is as close to instant gratification as you're going to get in getting fit. There will be an immediate increase in your muscle strength and endurance when you begin to exercise. An improvement can be felt and measured in just a few sessions. Significant improvement in strength and endurance, however, requires at least a month and a half. Once you get going, some regular exercise should be part of a lifelong routine.

HOW FAST DO YOU LIFT IT? Slowly. You don't get more benefit out of the exercise by lifting the resistance quickly. In fact, you could wind up getting no benefit at all if a weight speeding out of control uses your head as an impact attenuator—which for those of you not familiar with road safety nomenclature is one of those barrels of sand or big plastic accordions placed on highways to reduce the impact of an errant car.

In a shortening contraction of the muscle, increased speed decreases its lifting ability and therefore your maximum lift would be less, requiring more repetitions and more sets and more times a day and more times a week—you get the picture. So go slowly.

In isokinetic exercise, however, speed is everything. The specifics of isokinetic exercise will be discussed later, but it should be kept in mind that as opposed to isotonics, speed is the essence of isokinetic exercise. The muscle can be trained to improve in strength and endurance while moving at varying velocities. This is especially helpful in athletic training where specific muscle requirements can be matched up to individual sports.

SHOULD YOU CHANGE THE AMOUNT OF RESISTANCE WHEN MOVING? It makes sense to have different degrees of resistance through the range of movement of your exercise. Muscles and the joints they're trying to move have certain positions in which they can exert more force. For example, if your elbow is straight and you're trying to bend it to lift a ten-pound weight, it might be too much for you. If however, the elbow is already slightly bent, then ten pounds might be quite easy and not your maximum lift.

To make allowances for the differing strength of muscles in various joint positions, several exercise devices have been developed. These machines change the amount of weight that you're lifting as you move through the exercise. Again using the elbow as an example, the weight might start out at five pounds with the elbow straight, move up to eight pounds with the elbow bent halfway, and back down to five pounds with full bending. This way the muscle has the chance of being maximally loaded at various positions. Keep in mind that we're talking about isotonic resistive exercises. This concern is eliminated with isokinetic exercises where speed is constant, and you supply your own resistance by how great an effort you make. Your body makes an automatic adjustment because the muscle maintaining the same speed will not be able to push as hard at the beginning and end of the movement. This way the muscle has a maximum workout at every point from straight to fully bent elbow. Unfortunately isokinetic equipment is expensive and not generally for home use.

CHAPTER 8 SUMMARY: The amount of weight should be built up gradually and generally shouldn't be greater than what you can lift ten times in a row. In isotonics, move at a comfortable speed; in isokinetics move as fast as you can. A good routine would include five sets of five repetitions, but reach this goal gradually. Plan on an improvement in just a few sessions and a big change in a month and a half.

CHAPTER 9

ISOTONIC EXERCISES

Now that the whats and whys of isotonics are out of the way, it's time for the hows. Depending on your present degree of laziness and unfitness, some isotonics might be better for you than others. To make it easier for you to choose, the exercises have been graded by level of difficulty and how much effort is required to perform them.

TO RECAP SOME IMPORTANT POINTS:

1. You have a variety of options when it comes to equipment. You can use no weights, free weights, rubber tubing, or exercise machines to provide resistance for your isotonic exercise.

2. You're going to exercise only to 75 percent of your maximum potential.

3. Your sets and repetitions are going to be five and five, done slowly.

4. Every other day will be your goal for at least one and a half months.

And with that in mind, let the games begin.

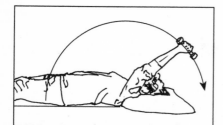

FIGURE 44

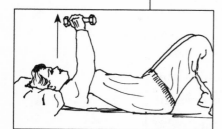

FIGURE 45

FIGURE 46

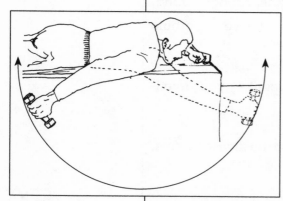

FIGURE 47

SHOULDERS

WITH OR WITHOUT WEIGHTS

1. Lie on your back with your hands at your sides, holding a weight. Keeping your arm straight, lift the weight back over your head as far as you can. Avoid any shoulder discomfort. Build up to 5 sets of 5 repetitions then increase the weights. Remember to exercise both arms. (See figure 44.)

2. Still on your back holding your weight, bend your elbow and keep it resting on the bed until your hand is aiming directly at the ceiling. Now push your hand up and try and touch the ceiling. Repeat. Avoid any shoulder discomfort. Build up to 5 sets of 5 repetitions then increase the weights. Exercise both arms. (See figure 45.)

3. Again on your back with your elbow resting on the bed, move your elbow out away from your body. The elbow can be anyplace between your side up to being even with your shoulder. Now bend your elbow so that your hand with the weight is toward the ceiling. Avoid any discomfort. Lower the weight forward to the bed, then back straight up, then lower the weight backward as far as you can. Keep repeating as you build up to 5 sets of 5 repetitions. (See figure 46.)

4. Lie stomach down on your bed with one arm over the edge holding a weight at your side. Move your hand down from your side toward the floor and up toward your head.

Avoid any shoulder discomfort. Build up to 5 sets of 5 repetitions then increase the weights. Remember to exercise both arms. (See figure 47.)

WITH RUBBER TUBING: Tie your tubing so that there is a sturdy loop on one end.

1. Securely fasten one end of your tubing to something like a door handle. Stand up and hold the unlooped end with your hand at your side while facing the door handle. Position yourself so that there is no slack in the tubing and pull back keeping your arm straight. Make sure you stand erect. Build up to 5 sets of 5 repetitions, then start to increase resistance, either stretch the tubing more tightly before you begin or add another tube. Remember to exercise both arms. (See figure 48.)

2. Turn so that your back is to the door handle. Have your hand at your side with the tubing stretched behind you without any slack. Keep your arm straight and lift your hand towards your face to shoulder level only. Build up to 5 sets of 5 repetitions, then start with the tubing more tightly stretched before you begin to exercise or add another tube. (See figure 49.)

3. Now stand sideways with your elbow at your side and the hand holding the tube toward the door. Hold the elbow you'll be exercising at your side with the other hand. Position yourself to take up the slack, then bring the hand holding the tube across your body until you touch the opposite elbow. Your arms will then be crossed on your stomach. Build up to 5 sets of 5 repetitions, then start with

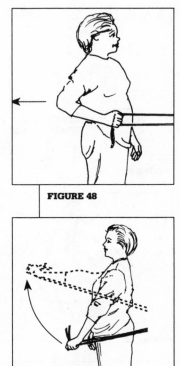

FIGURE 48

FIGURE 49

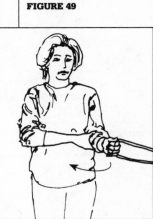

FIGURE 50

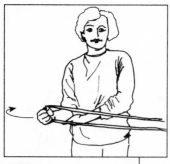

FIGURE 51

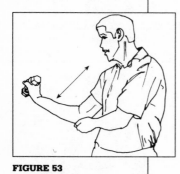

FIGURE 52

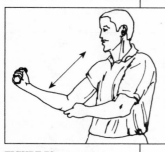

FIGURE 53

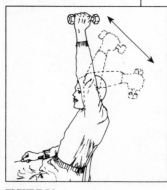

FIGURE 54

the tubing more tightly stretched before you begin to exercise, or you can add another tube. (See figure 50.)

4. Still holding the tube, turn around and face the other way with your arms crossed on your stomach and your hands touching your elbows. The tube should be stretched straight out from one hand toward the door. If there's any slack, move back until the tubing is taut. Move the tube across and then away from your body. Keep your elbow at the same angle and your forearm parallel to the floor. Build up to 5 sets of 5 repetitions. Increase your resistance either by pulling the tubing tighter or adding another one. (See figure 51.)

ARMS

WITH OR WITHOUT WEIGHTS

1. Stand or sit straight while holding the back of your exercising elbow with your other hand to keep the elbow slightly in front of your body. Hold the weight in your hand or wrap it around your wrist. Bend the elbow with the palm facing up and then lower it. This will exercise your biceps muscle. Build up to 5 sets of 5 repetitions, then add additional weight. (See figure 52.)

2. Do the same exercise only this time have your palm facing down. A different muscle is used. (See figure 53.)

Repeat your current number of sets and repetitions.

3. Now keep holding your weight and stretch your hand up over your head toward the ceiling. Stop if you have shoulder pain. With your arm up, let the elbow bend. As you repeatedly straighten and bend your

elbow, you'll be exercising the muscles on the back of your elbow, the triceps. (See figure 54.)

Repeat your current number of sets and repetitions.

WITH RUBBER TUBING

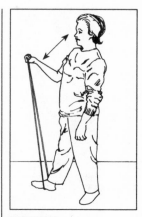

FIGURE 55

1. Securely place your foot in the loop on the end of your tube and stand on it. Keep the tube on the same side as the arm you're exercising. With your arm straight down at your side, take up any slack in the tube by wrapping the tube around your hand. Hold the back of your elbow with the other hand to keep your exercising elbow slightly in front of your body. Now pull up on the tube to bend your elbow, keeping your palm face up. Build up to 5 sets of 5 repetitions, after which you can stretch the tubing tighter or add another tube to increase resistance.(See figure 55.)

2. In the same position, turn your palm down, then follow the same procedure as above to exercise a different muscle in your elbow. Repeat your current number of sets and repetitions. (See figure 56.)

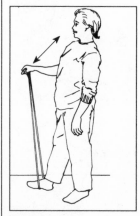

FIGURE 56

3. Hang the tube over the top of the door with the loop end on the far side. Shut the door. Your tube will now be hanging down from the top of the door. Stand with your back to the door and hold the tube in your hand as it comes over your shoulder. Take up the slack by wrapping it around your hand. Your elbow should be fully bent with the hand holding the tube up near your shoulder. Straighten your elbow as much as you can for the required number of sets. You'll be strengthening the muscle on the back of the arm, the triceps. (See figure 57.)

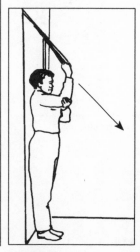

FIGURE 57

WRISTS

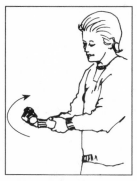

FIGURE 58

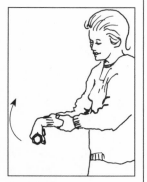

FIGURE 59

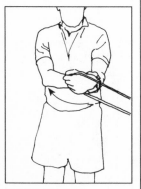

FIGURE 60

WITH OR WITHOUT WEIGHTS

1. Use a very light weight for the wrists. Start with 1 pound. Stand or sit with your elbow in at your side and your palm out as if you were accepting change from a purchase. Support the wrist with your other hand. Slowly bend your wrist so that your palm moves more toward the ceiling. Repeat 5 times and build up to your current number of sets and repetitions. (See figure 58.)

2. Then in the same position with your elbow bent at your side, turn your palm toward the floor while holding the weight and lift the back of your hand up toward the ceiling. Repeat the usual 5 repetitions and slowly build up the number of sets. (See figure 59.)

These exercises are particularly useful in maintaining strong forearms and can help you avoid the dreaded golf and tennis elbows.

WITH RUBBER TUBING

1. Stand sideways to the door with the tube wrapped around your hand and your palm facing in toward your body. Hold your wrist with the other hand. Keeping the wrist steady, pull the tube so that your palm moves toward your body. (See figure 60.)

Build up to 5 sets of 5 repetitions, then start with the tubing more tightly stretched before you begin to exercise or add another tube.

2. Turn and face the opposite direction so that you'll have to bend your wrist backwards to pull the tube. Remember to keep your wrist steady by holding it with the other hand.

Repeat your current number of sets and repetitions. (See figure 61.)

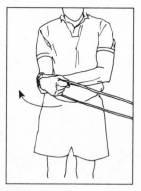

FIGURE 61

BACK

WITH—BUT MOSTLY WITHOUT—WEIGHTS

Two major muscle groups required for a strong back are the abdominal or stomach muscles and the extensors or back muscles. The abdominal muscles serve to support the spine from the front of your body. Well-conditioned stomach muscles are very important in supporting the lower back, which is under great strain most of the time from poor posture, prolonged sitting in a slumped position (like reading or watching TV in bed), and bending from the waist to reach the floor. The extensors or back muscles serve to maintain your spine in an erect and straight position.

The exercises for both of these groups usually don't require weights. Your muscles have quite a load just raising your body from the waist up, which constitutes about 40 percent of your total body weight. So a 185-pound person doing a sit-up or back extensions on his stomach could be lifting 74 pounds. Who needs penny rolls when you're trying to toss around that much weight? We have one thing to confess. The back exercises offered here are classics. They're good for the Lazy Person and Any Person and will be found in nearly ever exercise program. Don't forget to breathe by counting out loud.

IF YOU HAVE LOWER BACK PROBLEMS, CONSULT YOUR PHYSICIAN OR PHYSICAL THERAPIST BEFORE DOING THESE EXERCISES.

METHOD:

1. To strengthen back muscles, lie on your stomach, arms at your sides. Lift your shoulders and head up from the bed and hold. Keep the neck straight, don't bend your head back.

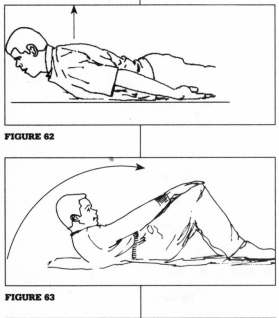

FIGURE 62

FIGURE 63

You only have to raise up several inches to achieve the desired effect. Slowly (count out loud "One thousand one, one thousand two, one thousand three") repeat the lift 5 times. Build up to your required number of sets. (See figure 62.)

2. To strengthen your stomach muscles, lie on your back with knees bent and feet on the bed or floor (don't hook your feet under anything). Stretch your arms out straight toward your bent knees and try and touch your knees by lifting your head and shoulders up from the floor. Repeat 5 times, if you're able. Gradually build up to performing several sets of this exercise. (See figure 63.)

3. When you're able to perform 5 sets of 5 repetitions of the above exercise, you can make it more difficult by crossing your arms on your chest instead of having your arms stretched out toward your knees. (See figure 64.)

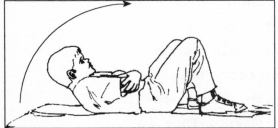

FIGURE 64

WITH RUBBER TUBING (This isn't the easiest thing to set up, but you might want to try.)

1. If you have a long enough piece of elastic or rubber tubing, you can loop it around your chest and then securely

fasten the other end of the tubing to a doorknob. To keep the loop from slipping off, hook it onto the knob on the back of the door and then shut the door. Either sitting or standing, lean forward or backward trying to stretch the tubing. Stop your pull forward or backward after your head has moved about twelve inches. As you lean forward, you'll be strengthening your stomach muscles. As you lean backwards, you'll be firming up your back muscles. Move both ways slowly throughout the stretch and repeat 5 times. Take your time building up to 5 sets of 5 repetitions. (See figure 65.) Remember to avoid pain with any of these back exercises!!

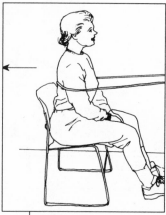

FIGURE 65

HIPS

WITH OR WITHOUT WEIGHTS

Hip muscles move the leg in just about any direction in relation to your pelvis. However, there are considerable limits on this motion compared with the very flexible shoulder. As a trade-off for limited motion, the hip is very sturdy and stable. While the hip can perform many different motions by combining different muscle groups, we'll stay with four directions: forward, backward, in, and out. If you have two weights, you can attach them to both left and right legs *above the knee* and do both hips at once.

1. FORWARD: Lie on your back and attach a weight to the leg that you'll be exercising (1 or 2 pounds is fine). Keep the other knee bent with the foot on the floor to protect your lower back. Lift the leg with the weight straight up about 1

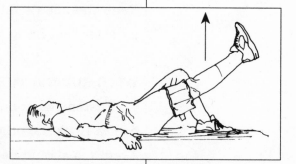

FIGURE 66

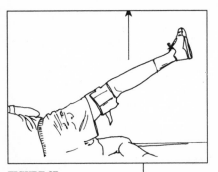

FIGURE 67

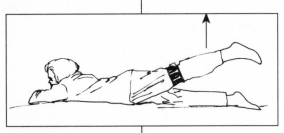

FIGURE 68

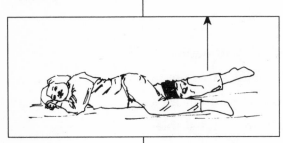

FIGURE 69

1/2 feet from the floor. Repeat 5 times and slowly build your sets to 5. (See figure 66.)

2. OUT: Roll a quarter turn onto the side without the weight. Make sure your body is straight (perpendicular) and not leaning forward or backward. Use a hand to keep straight. Lift the top leg with the weight toward the ceiling about 1 and 1/2 feet. Repeat 5 times and slowly increase sets. (See figure 67.)

3. BACKWARD: Roll onto your stomach. Lift one leg at a time up from the bed. If you have a weight on each leg, do one leg at a time. Keep the knee straight. This strengthens the buttock muscles. Repeat 5 times for each set. (See figure 68.)

4. IN: And now onto your other side. The leg to exercise is closest to the floor. Cross the leg that you're not exercising over the bottom leg and out of the way. The object is to lift the bottom leg up off the floor. Keep the knee straight. This strengthens the inner thigh or muscles that bring the hip in. (See figure 69.)

WITH RUBBER TUBING

Fasten the tubing to a sturdy table that will not move easily. Hook the other end of the tubing to your ankle. These exercises should be done standing. Have something nearby to hold for balance. For added difficulty, don't hold on and

114

discover what a great workout this is for the leg that's not stretching the tube.

1. FORWARD: With the tube around your ankle stretching out behind you, keep your knee straight and move your leg forward like you were trying to step over a puddle. Repeat 5 times. Build up the sets slowly. (See figure 70.)

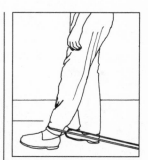

FIGURE 70

2. IN: Make a 1/4 turn so that the tube is stretched from the table to your nearest leg. Move the leg slightly forward, and then pull the leg with the tube across the front of the other leg, as if you were trying to cross your legs. Repeat 5 times. (See figure 71.)

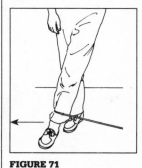

FIGURE 71

3. BACKWARD: Again make a 1/4 revolution so that the tube is stretched out in front of you. Pull your leg backwards with the knee straight. Repeat 5 times for each set. (See figure 72.)

4. OUT: Turn your body the last 1/4 turn, so that the tube is stretched across in front of you. Move the leg with the tube slightly forward so the tube doesn't hit the other leg. In a scissor motion, stretch your leg out to the side. Repeat 5 times. (See figure 73.)

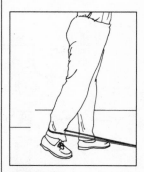

FIGURE 72

KNEES

WITH OR WITHOUT WEIGHTS

The two major muscle groups that control the knee—the quadriceps on top of your thigh and the hamstrings on the back—are understandably very strong since they're essential for walking, running, climbing stairs, playing a game, etc. A common computerized test to determine the strength of the quadriceps muscle shows that in-shape athletes can pro-

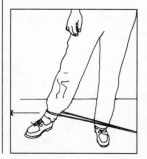

FIGURE 73

duce a torque equal to their own body weight with just one leg. So that if they weigh 200 pounds, they should be able to produce 200 foot-pounds of torque. Most of us are probably in the 50 percent range versus our body weight. The quadriceps, however, build up very quickly, and you'll notice almost immediate changes in the shape and strength of your thighs after performing these exercises.

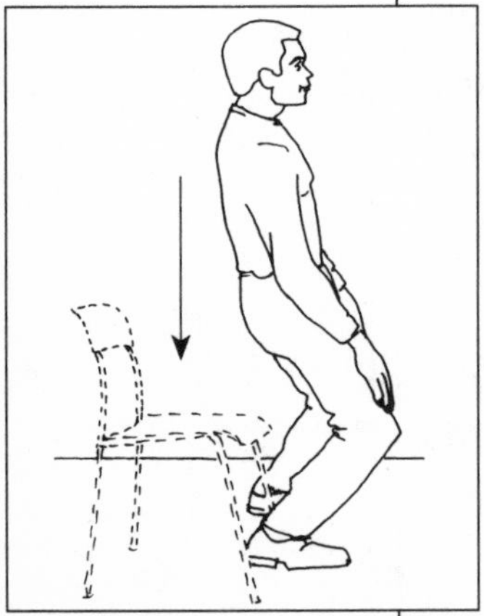

QUADRICEPS:

1. The modified squat is one of the best exercises to increase quad strength. Stand with your feet apart, toes slightly pointed out. Keep your low back straight and begin to slowly bend your knees as if you were going to sit on a chair. Keep your heels on the ground, and don't let your kneecaps go past an imaginary line coming straight up from your toes. Go up and down slowly, 3 seconds each way and go no lower than if you were sitting on a chair. Repeat 5 times and slowly build up to 5 sets. To make this more difficult, you can hold a weight, but in most cases an easier way is to exercise only one leg at a time. This is most easily done while standing sideways on a stairstep or on a large telephone book. (See figure 74.)

2. You can also strengthen the quads by adding *ankle*, instead of above-the-knee, weights to the hip exercises that were described above. We start with two. (See figure 75.)

3. Forward—Lie on your back with one knee bent and the foot resting on the bed or floor. Attach your ankle weight (usually a pound or two

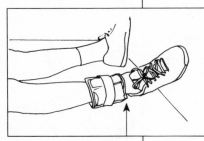

FIGURE 74

FIGURE 75

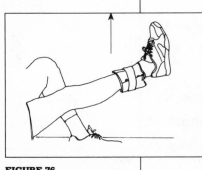

FIGURE 76

to begin) to the other leg which is straight out. Have the toes slightly pointed outward. Slowly lift the leg straight up approximately one foot from the surface and hold for a 5 count. Repeat 5 times and slowly build up to 5 sets. (See figure 76.)

4. Next, stay in the same position but slightly bend the knee of the straight leg with the weight on the ankle. Then proceed to lift for 5 times with a 5 count at the top. Build up to 5 sets. This exercise will be slightly more difficult than with the leg straight. (See figure 77.)

5. A very easy exercise for the quadriceps is to sit on a high chair or stool and slowly straighten your knee—but *not totally*! Lift only about 2/3 of the way up. Repeat 5 times and slowly build up to 5 sets with a 5 count at the top. (See figure 78.)

6. Next in the same seated position, fully straighten one knee. Then let it bend so that your foot lowers toward the floor a few inches, hold for a 5 count and then fully straighten again and repeat. These seated exercises cover the full range of motion of the knee but prevent any irritation to your kneecap. (See figure 79.)

7. Add one or two pound ankle weights to the above exercises when ready. (See figure 80.)

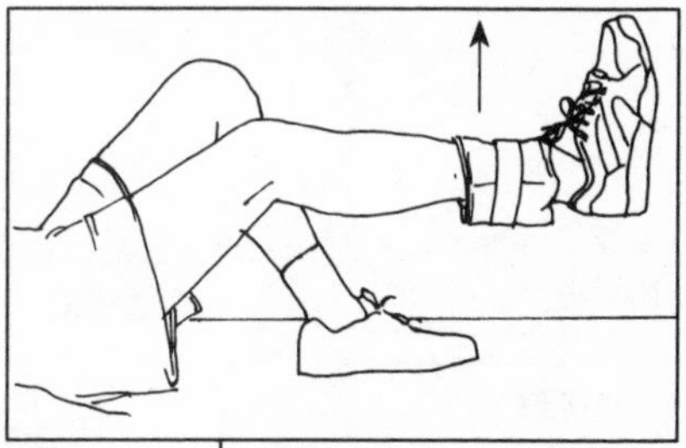

HAMSTRINGS:

1. Lie on your stomach and bend one knee, lifting your foot up from the floor or bed. You should lift high enough so that the sole of the foot is pointing upwards toward the ceil-

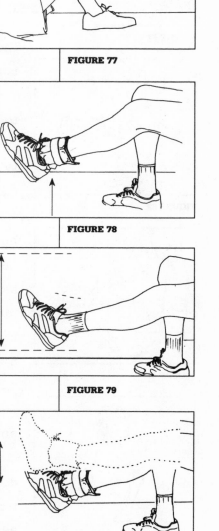

FIGURE 77

FIGURE 78

FIGURE 79

FIGURE 80

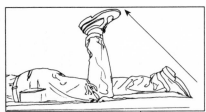

FIGURE 81

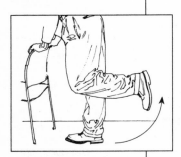

FIGURE 82

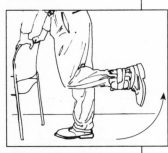

FIGURE 83

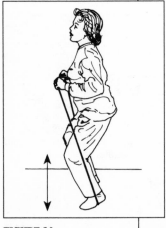

FIGURE 84

ing. Five sets of five with a five count at the top should do it. (See figure 81.)

2. Stand, holding onto the back of a chair, and again bend one knee until the sole of the foot is pointing straight backwards (a 90 degree angle at the knee). Do 5 sets of 5 with a 5 count when your knee is fully bent. (See figure 82.)

Add ankle weights (one or two pounds) when ready to the above exercises. (See figure 83.)

WITH RUBBER TUBING

QUADRICEPS:

1. Stand on the middle of your length of tubing and hold an end in each hand with arms straight. Slightly bend your knees and then take up the slack in the tubing. This is a simple, effective way to add some resistance to a modified squat exercise. Straighten your knees while holding the tubing tight. Repeat 5 times for 5 sets with a 5 count at the top when the knees are straight. (See figure 84.)

2. Stand or sit with the tubing around your ankle and secured behind you (for example, tied to a sturdy chair leg) then move your leg forward. When sitting, don't completely straighten the leg. Take it up about two-thirds of the way. You can also exercise the quads as described above while sitting with the knee straight and bending it just slightly, take up the slack in the tubing, and then straighten. Repeat 5 times for 5 sets with a 5 count when the tubing is under tension. (See figure 85.)

HAMSTRINGS:

1. Stand or sit with the tubing looped around the back of your ankle and securely fastened in front of you. Pull back to bend your knee. Repeat 5 times for 5 sets with a 5 count when the tubing is under tension. (See figure 86.)

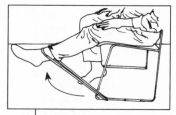

FIGURE 85

ANKLES

WITH OR WITHOUT WEIGHTS

CALF:

1. Rise up on your toes. If you're not ready for the Bolshoi, holding on for balance is perfectly all right. This is very simple to do anyplace, at home, in an elevator, or at the office. To increase the effort, hold one foot off the floor so you're rising up on just one leg. This exercise is excellent on long plane or train rides to prevent swelling in your legs and stiffness. Tensing the calf muscles pumps the blood in your leg so that your veins can return blood to your heart. Fainting on the parade ground was often attributed to blood pooling in the legs and shortchanging the brain. Occasionally tightening the calves even though "at attention" prevents hitting the deck. Begin with 5 repetitions and a pause at the top for a 5 count, then build up to 5 sets. (See figure 87.)

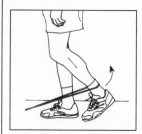

FIGURE 86

2. For more difficult toe raises, stand on a step with your heel hanging over the edge. Hold the railing for balance. Let your heel drop below the step, then rise up until you're on your toes. (See figure 88.)

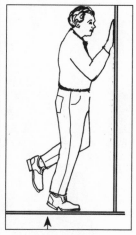

FIGURE 87

OTHER ANKLE MUSCLES:

In either a seated position or with your legs out straight:

1. Lift your foot up so that the top of your ankle moves

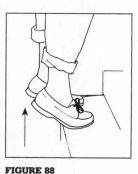

FIGURE 88

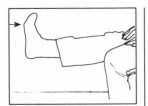

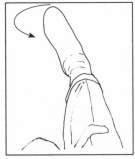

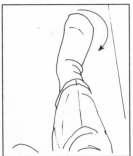

FIGURE 89

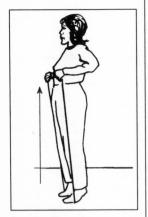

FIGURE 90

toward your face; 2. Turn your foot in so that the instep is facing the other leg; 3. Turn your foot out so that the instep faces away from the other leg. Begin with 5 repetitions and a pause after moving for a 5 count, then build up to 5 sets. (See figure 89.)

For more resistance, do the above exercises with a weight strapped around your toes.

WITH RUBBER TUBING

CALF:

1. Stand on the center of your tubing and hold the two ends tight. Push up on your toes to stretch the tubing, and you'll be doing resistive exercise. (See figure 90.)

2. Alternately, sit down with your leg out straight and the tubing looped around your foot. Hold the two ends and push down like you were stepping on a gas pedal. (See figure 91.)

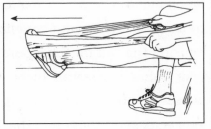

FIGURE 91

Repeat both of these 5 times building up to 5 sets and hold for a count of 5 when you push.

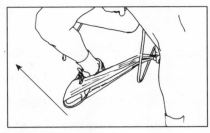

FIGURE 92

OTHER ANKLE MUSCLES:

1. Sit in a chair or stand and loop the tubing around the outside of your foot. Securely fasten the tubing and try to turn your foot out away from the other leg. (See figure 92.)

2. Loop the tubing around the inside of your foot with the ends out away from the foot. Then turn your foot in toward the other foot. (See figure 93.)

3. Loop the tubing around the top of your foot, and then lift your foot.

Some of these other ankle exercises can be done with the tubing held by the other foot or fastened to something secure. Repeat these 5 times building up to 5 sets and hold for a count of 5 when you push. (See figure 94.)

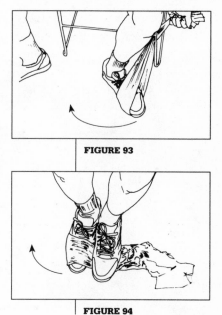

FIGURE 93

FIGURE 94

CHAPTER 10

AEROBIC EXERCISE

In addition to developing muscles that are both flexible, strong, in good condition, and have good endurance, you need to develop your heart and lungs. That's where aerobic exercise comes in.

The heart is a muscle that can be strengthened just like any other by using it. If the heart is strong, it's able to provide your body with the oxygen it needs to function with less effort. Your breathing is regular, and you don't start panting when you lean down to pick up a pencil from the floor. There is a greater capacity for doing the things you want to do. Sports are easier to play, and generally you have better endurance when performing any task.

Some champion athletes have very low heart rates, or beats per minutes, when they're resting. The great tennis star, Bjorn Borg, was said to have a resting heart rate of thirty-five, which means his heart only had to beat thirty-five times per minute to supply his body with oxygen while at rest.

More common folk have average heart rates of around seventy. So when Borg was playing flat out in a tie breaker against Jimmy Connors, his heart rate—even though it had doubled to get more oxygen to his muscles—would have been the same as the average person's when sitting still. Someone who started at seventy-two beats per minute and required extra oxygen for increased muscle activity would quickly be up to more than one hundred beats per minute.

There are calculations for the upper limits of our heart rate and are based on age, weight, and general condition. It's easy to see that a strong heart that can provide the necessary oxygen with fewer beats per minute has a much larger reserve and can provide more energy without straining. Over the course of a day, a week, a year, the heart will beat many thousands of time less if it's strong.

Your physician may advise you to have a stress test. In this test, usually on a treadmill, you're required to walk faster and faster. More oxygen has to get to your muscles, especially those in your legs, therefore your heart has to beat faster.

Measurements can be made of how much oxygen you're using, that is, how efficiently your heart and muscles are working, and potential heart problems may be uncovered by a careful analysis of the way your heart beats (by means of an electrocardiogram).

Bill Rodgers, the great American marathon runner, was being complimented by a reporter for winning the twenty-six-mile race in a little more than two hours. As they were standing at the finishing line, other entrants were crossing it, clocking in at three, four, and even five hours. When asked about these late finishers, Rodgers expressed the utmost admiration for being able to run for five hours. He didn't feel he could possibly run that long, which was why he ran the race in only two.

Even though his comment was a bit tongue-in-cheek, the point is well taken and applies to the discussion of aerobic exercise. The strong heart and lungs can more easily supply oxygen to the muscles being using without straining or beating too fast. Rodgers was able to keep his leg muscles working vigorously without overtaxing his heart and so finished in two hours.

By performing aerobic exercise, or carefully overloading the demands on the heart, the heart becomes stronger. Just as muscles are overloaded or stressed by lifting weights or pulling tubing, aerobic exercise does the same for the heart. Muscles also benefit from aerobics. To increase the demand on the heart, you have to do some sort of activity in which muscles are used. Use increases strength and conditioning.

There are several formulas for calculating how much you should overload your heart to obtain the benefits of aerobic exercise. In *young and healthy persons*, subtract your age from 220 and then aim for between 60 and 80 percent of that number for your target rate.

For example, if you're a healthy twenty year old, the calculation would be:

	220		220	
	—20 years old		—20 years old	
	200		200	
	x .60		x .80	
between	120	and	160	target beats per minute

THIS FORMULA ABSOLUTELY DOES NOT APPLY TO MIDDLE AGED AND OLDER PEOPLE OR TO THOSE WITH A HEALTH PROBLEM. YOUR TARGET RATE SHOULD BE DETERMINED BY A HEALTH PROFESSIONAL AFTER CAREFUL ANALYSIS!!!!

If you're interested in heart rate targets, between 60 percent and 80 percent of capacity by age, refer back to the table on page 35. The Lazy Person's way is to start at 60 percent. If you wish to have a greater effect later, you can work up toward 80 percent gradually.

There are many devices available for measuring your heart rate. They attach to your ear or hand and will show you the beats per minute of your heart. You can also take your pulse in the manner described on pages 34-35.

Once you get to your target heart rate, the exercise should continue for twenty to thirty minutes. Of course, that's after you've built up to that time over several months, starting from sixty seconds and adding thirty seconds a day.

Remember, the Lazy Person's credo is still in effect. If you don't feel like working out for twenty or thirty minutes, okay. You don't have to, but do *something*. Something is better than nothing. Anything you do regularly is better than the ideal exercise you don't do at all. Conversely, if you wish to build up slowly to forty-five minutes of exercise a day or even one hour, this shouldn't hurt if you've built up slowly and you don't have a physical condition or illness that precludes it.

Recent studies and recommendations advise exercising aerobically on a daily basis. Previously three or four times per week was thought to be adequate. We recommend aerobic exercising five or six days a week. The body needs some time to recover. If you're over thirty-five, you shouldn't do the same aerobic exercise every day, but rather switch off between different ones. This is especially true if you run or jog, or do something else that is hard on the joints, like tennis or racquetball. Exercises that are very gentle on the joints, like ski machines or bicycling, could be done five or six days a week.

Your aerobic exercise should be divided into three phases: 1) the warm-up, which gets the muscles and entire body ready to increase the heart rate, and should be at least five minutes; 2) the aerobic part, where you aim for your target rate and keep it there for thirty minutes, once you've built up your endurance; 3) and lastly, the cool-down.

The warm-up is used to get blood flowing through the muscles thereby, surprise, surprise, warming them up. This is akin to starting a car on a cold day when the oil in the engine is thick and needs to be heated enough so that the metal parts work smoothly and efficiently.

A warm-up also allows for changes in your nerves which can then alert the breathing muscles that some exercise will begin shortly. The muscles and joints also have a chance to loosen up and prepare for the impending exertion.

You should warm up gradually with gentle stretches, some calisthenics (many of the exercises talked about earlier in the book are good to do), and perhaps light jogging in place. You shouldn't be fatigued at all by performing the warm-up, and your heart rate should increase to within twenty beats of your target rate. If your target rate is 110 beats per minute, then the warm-up should bring you to a pulse of about 90. Once you have increased your aerobic exercise time to 30 minutes, then the warm-up should be about *10 minutes*.

You can warm up with the same aerobic exercise you'll be doing that day, only do it slower. However, it's good to gradually stretch the muscles further than the movement required for your aerobic exercise.

Once you've gotten your blood moving, it's time for the aerobic part of your workout. You know your target rate ahead of time, and you're monitoring your pulse. When you reach your target rate, start the clock on your aerobic workout. You should take your pulse every minute when you're a beginner. Later on, when you have a sense of how hard you're working, you can increase the time between pulse checks to two, three, and even five minutes.

The effort should be to use the large muscle groups (like the buttocks, calves, and thighs) in a repetitive way to raise the pulse while the muscles use up oxygen in the blood, the essence of aerobic exercise. There are several ways to go about doing the program. The exercise can be *continuous*, *intervals*, *circuit*, or a *combination of circuit and intervals*. Each has advantages and disadvantages.

Continuous aerobic training is fairly self-explanatory but requires the best conditioning and probably shouldn't be tried by the Lazy Person until a fairly consistent routine is established. The task which you're performing—walking, riding a bike, jogging, cross-country skiing, or whatever—should be done continuously at a degree of difficulty so that your pulse stays at your target level. This greatly improves your endurance for those ten-mile treks in the great outdoors of the Tibetan mountains.

Interval training is quite popular now and builds up strength. In fact, you can perform more work in total by taking little rests than by working continuously. So as you might have guessed, interval training is done by either resting totally or by slowing down every few minutes. There are various formulas for calculating the length of the work/rest intervals, but an easy one is 1 to 3. So if you were walking, walk quickly for fifteen seconds, then slow your pace for the next forty-five seconds. Keep repeating this one-minute routine. You can perform these intervals doing almost any activity.

Circuit training requires some imagination and planning. The exercises are varied and should include both aerobic exercise and the strengthening exercises described earlier with tubing, weights, or isometrics (making a muscle). To get a good workout you have to keep on the go and have an activity ready one after the other.

The last type of aerobic exercise is a combination of circuit and interval. This method puts rest or slow-down periods in the circuit which allows you to use all aspects of the muscle, both with oxygen being demanded and without.

The third and last phase of the exercise is the cool-down. At last! Basically you do the same as the warm-up for five to ten minutes to allow the muscles and joints to slowly return to their preexercise condition. So after walking briskly around the block, you shouldn't flop on the couch and cool down by hefting the remote control. Rather walk slowly and stretch a bit for another five minutes after your brisk walk.

There are many benefits to an aerobic program. Breathing is easier, the heart works better, circulation is improved, muscles have more flexibility and strength, and there's a general sense of well-being.

Don't forget that sex is an excellent aerobic exercise. Depending on whether you're on top, how active you are, and how long your lovemaking lasts, you can burn from fifty to three hundred calories in one session. And who said exercise has to be boring?

Remember there is a noted paradox in the body-mind relationship in that meditation (relaxation) is good for the body and exercise is good for the mind. Of course, this body-mind relationship is not one or the other—both are beneficial for YOU.

CHAPTER 11

HOME EXERCISE

It has become increasingly popular to exercise at home. This is especially true for the Lazy Person. Sometimes the effort to change and travel back and forth to a gym is too much. Even if you do go to a gym regularly, you may want something to do on off days when you're home. Many of the exercises described earlier require little if any equipment. Just a few pounds of weights and/or some elastic tubing or just your own body weight properly used.

There may come a point, however, when even a Lazy Person like you might want to expand your possibilities beyond penny rolls and rubber bands. Yes, you might want expend the energy of opening your wallet and buying some pieces of home equipment. Even if you never actually use them, they make excellent clothes hangers.

An all-time favorite for home use is the stationary bike. It can have a reading stand on the handlebars and be placed anywhere, including in front of the tube. The wheel in front is usually metal and should be quite heavy to provide a smooth, even ride. The kind that works on air resistance works well too. The seat should be easily adjustable and comfortable. No need for the "Tour de France" three-inch-wide pie-shaped seat. It would also be nice for the pedals to have toe loops to make it easier to keep your foot in place. You might also think about getting a bike with easily adjusted pedaling resistance, an RPM (revolutions per minute) meter, an odometer (to determine how far you would have gone if you were indeed going anyplace), and a timer.

The stationary bike provides resistive exercise for the legs as well as aerobic exercise for the heart and lungs. Again, we can't emphasize enough that before beginning any aerobic activity for the first time in awhile, you should be given a clean bill of health by your physician.

It's a must that you proceed slowly. You should begin with only one minute on the bike with little if any resistance to pedaling. The seat should be adjusted high enough so that your knee is just slightly bent when the pedal is at the bottom of its circle. The RPMs or times you complete a full turn of the pedals in a minute should not be greater than fifty or sixty. Don't worry about progressing too slowly. If you add thirty seconds to your exercise time each session, you'll be up to twenty or thirty minutes in no time at all.

The amount of effort you expend should be based on your original condition, health status, age, and goals. And again, it would be the best of all worlds if you worked out aerobically five or six times a week. Since we all know that the best of all worlds isn't always where we live, do it as often as you can.

Since, stationary bikes vary greatly in price, it pays to shop around with the above considerations in mind. For the budget conscious, bikes seem to be one of the mainstays of Saturday morning yard or apartment sales. See if you can't pick up a good used one.

Another very popular piece of equipment for the home is the cross-country skiing machine. These caught on several years ago and have proven to be one of the best forms of exercise for the whole body. Arms and legs are exercised and unlike a rowing machine, you're benefiting by using the additional muscles required to stand up. The equipment should be sturdy and have easily adjustable resistances for both arms and legs. For those not so coordinated or wanting to exercise only the legs or only the arms, the machine should work independently for either arms or legs. One of the skiing machine's big advantages for the Lazy Person is you don't have to lift your feet. Just think of it, all the exercise you could ever want without even lifting your feet, right in the comfort of your own home.

The ski machines like the stationary bikes vary greatly in cost. Plan to spend several hundred dollars, however, to get a quality piece of equipment that will last and provide a comfortable exercise session but not the thrill of falling in the snow or your apartment.

Depending on your budget and your inclination to exercise at home, there are, of course, many other pieces of exercise equipment, such as the treadmill. Treadmills can be great—if you can afford them. For one worth working out on, you have to figure on forking over a minimum of more than a thousand dollars. A really high-quality machine will set you back several thousand.

A new and very popular form of aerobic exercise is stepping. Stepping can be done either on boxes of varying heights or on a machine which simulates stair climbing. While these machines can provide a vigorous workout, caution is indicated to prevent knee irritation. Knees have just so many bends in them over a lifetime. Just as coaches have realized that the duckwalk (squatting down and scurrying along) wreaks havoc on the knees, so stepping on boxes or using a stair-climbing machine can cause trouble. If the knees bend more than twenty degrees, your kneecap may start protesting. If you do use boxes or a stair-climbing machine, limit the height of the step to no more than six inches.

As with any exercise equipment, follow the general guidelines of sturdiness, durability, and safety. Make sure any stair-climbing equipment you purchase will allow you to limit the distance the step moves as you go up.

Another general piece of equipment for the home would be some sort of combination or multiple station machine. Various exercises would be possible by altering or adjusting the machine. Upper body and lower body work is usually possible with many variations. There are also different methods of providing resistance to the individual exercises. Stacks of iron weights, thick rubber bands, and hydraulic tubes are just some of the methods used.

You want to get a device that's easy to set up as well as change to different exercises. If you're going to spend forty-five minutes and five bruised knuckles attempting to go from knee-straightening to knee-bending exercises, the machine will probably end up in your attic. Another consideration is the number of different exercises that can be performed on the machine. Do you really need—or want—to do five variations of the bench press or lat pulls? A simpler machine might be easier to set up, less expensive, and include all the various exercises that you plan to do. Shop around and visit a quality fitness equipment store where a knowledgeable sales person can direct you to something that fits your needs and budget.

There are many different types of individual exercise gadgets. Springs to squeeze, balls to throw, boards to balance on, seats to slide on, ad infinitum. Most offer some activity that can be beneficial if done safely, your expectations are not unreasonable, and you begin very, very slowly. Make sure to avoid pieces of equipment that guarantee "instant" results—as much as you might admire Suzanne Somers' thighs—or to remove fat from one particular part of the body.

CHAPTER 12

THE CHECKUP

All Lazy People—and that means you—should have a physical before beginning an aerobic exercise program. Many of the strengthening exercises can be done without first checking with your doctor if you carefully follow the instructions outlined earlier. If you have any reason to believe that the exercises could be a problem for you, then a checkup with your physician is in order. We don't want to sound like your crotchety old maid aunt, but it's especially important for those who might have high blood pressure, heart problems, severe arthritis, any major illness, or are taking medication. Once you have been cleared to exercise, it's crucial to begin slowly.

You might also consider making an appointment with a physical therapist. Therapists are trained to perform postural evaluations, grade your muscle strength and flexibility, determine your body fat percentage and your overall conditioning. They're also knowledgeable about particular diseases or illnesses that might require specific types of exercise. Therapists can evaluate your ability to perform a particular sport or activity and suggest an exercise program of stretching and strengthening to prepare you for the activity or better your participation.

CHAPTER 13

CHOOSING A FITNESS CENTER

There is a long-standing joke that at some of the "in" centers, you have to be in shape before you join. Our suggestions are for the Lazy Person just starting out who wants to do more than is available at home and has the commitment to take advantage of membership. Many of the fitness centers presume that a great number of annual memberships will drop out or underutilize the facility. Make sure that you want to visit regularly before you plunk down your money. Ask whether there's a trial membership. And don't let them bamboozle you into signing up for a year five minutes after you've walked in. Some fitness centers won't even be around that long.

Several years ago, Dave paid $500 for an annual membership in a local center mainly to use its Olympic-sized pool. In twelve months, he took exactly two dips. In other words, he paid $250 a dip.

Visit several fitness centers before you join. And be sure to go at about the same time of day that you intend to exercise. Right after the workday is usually quite crowded, and there could be a wait for a particular machine, or the track might look like a swarm of bees moving around an oval.

Some of the questions you want answered include whether you'll be prescreened to set up a program based on your fitness level. Is an orientation provided for each piece of equipment that you use? Is the staff qualified, and are they members of any exercise associations? Does the staff encourage and is there time for warm-up and cool-down periods? Are there easily used monitors for your pulse, and is the staff trained in CPR (cardiopulmonary resuscitation), although you fervently hope they'll never have to use it? What are the lockers like? Is there child care? (Of course, if you don't have a child, you skip that question.) Would you find the exercises reasonable for your level of fitness or are the classes better suited for Carl Lewis?

All these questions should be answered. And don't take someone else's word for it—go and see for yourself.

CHAPTER 14

SAMPLE PROGRAMS

O kay, dear Lazy Person, what you've been waiting for— sample programs. Keep in mind, these are samples. Your specific program depends on your specific goals. You may wish to do muscle-strengthening exercises to help your arthritis, or primarily aerobic exercises to help your weight control, or some combination of exercises. Your particular regimen should be one that meets your goals—that includes how much time you wish to spend. These samples just give you an idea of what some people do and what might be reasonable.

SAMPLE ISOMETRIC PROGRAM

The easiest program to begin is a group of isometric exercises. These can be done at anytime and virtually anyplace. Most people won't even realize that you're exercising—if you remember to count so you don't turn an unbecoming purple in the face. Try some or all of the exercise on page 144. Remember to hold for a count of 5 and perform 5 repetitions.

SAMPLE ISOTONIC PROGRAM

Another program that is easy to begin is a group of isotonic exercises. These can be done with little, if any, equipment. People around you will know that you're exercising when you start counting—and when you eventually take to boasting about the number of reps and sets you do. Try some or all of the exercise on page 145. Remember to perform 5 repetitions.

SAMPLE AEROBIC PROGRAM

If your goals are cardiovascular fitness, or weight control, or to decrease cholesterol, you may want to focus on aerobic exercise. A sample program would have you choose one or more aerobic exercises, such as bicycling (stationary and/or outdoor), running, jogging, racewalking, cross-country ski machine, stair-climbing, swimming, etc. Swimming doesn't help as much for weight control, but it will help you reach the other aerobic goals. If you're under thirty-five, you could focus on one exercise. If you're over thirty-five, or have joint problems, you should alternate exercises on different days and/or focus on exercises that aren't jarring to the joints, especially walking.

Warm up, doing either stretches and isotonics, or a slower version of the aerobic exercise you've chosen. Monitor your pulse and start counting your aerobic time when your pulse reaches 60 percent of your capacity (see table on page 35).

DAY	TIME
1	1 minute
2	90 seconds
3	2 minutes
4	2 minutes, 30 seconds
5	3 minutes
6	3 minutes, 30 seconds
7	rest

and so on.

You get the picture. Build up until you're at twenty or thirty minutes, or forty-five, or sixty, or whatever you desire. Remember, if you're injured or sick, restart as soon as you can, subtracting no time for up to three days off, and thirty seconds less exercise for every day more than three you haven't exercised.

SAMPLE ISOMETRIC PROGRAM

DIRECTIONS FOR EXERCISE

1. Push in the direction of arrow.
2. Do not allow any movement.
3. Keep pushing for 5 seconds.
4. Count out loud to 5.
5. Repeat above 5 times.
6. Do both sides of the body.
7. Stop if painful and consult a professional.

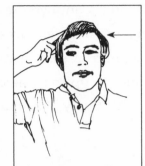

FIGURE 3—see page 79.

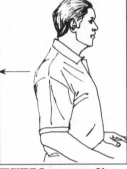

FIGURE 5—see page 81.

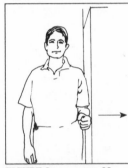

FIGURE 8—see page 82.

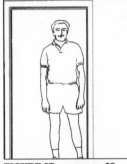

FIGURE 11—see page 83.

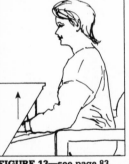

FIGURE 13—see page 83.

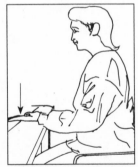

FIGURE 14—see page 84.

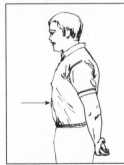

FIGURE 22—see page 87.

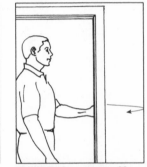

FIGURE 27—see page 89.

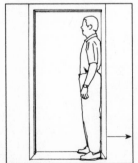

FIGURE 28—see page 89.

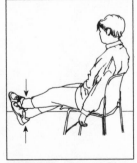

FIGURE 33—see page 91.

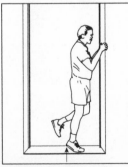

FIGURE 38—see page 93.

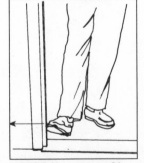

FIGURE 40—see page 94.

SAMPLE ISOTONIC PROGRAM

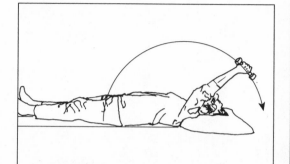

FIGURE 44—see page 106.

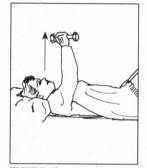

FIGURE 45—see page 106.

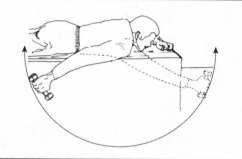

FIGURE 47—see page 106.

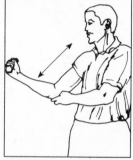

FIGURE 52—see page 108.

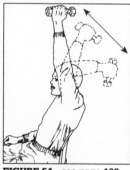

FIGURE 54—see page 108.

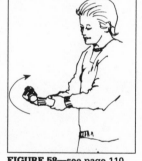

FIGURE 58—see page 110.

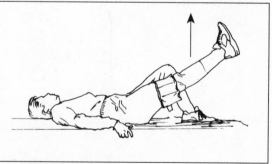

FIGURE 66—see page 113.

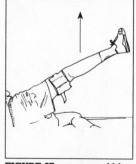

FIGURE 67—see page 114.

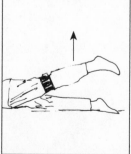

FIGURE 68—see page 114.

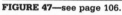

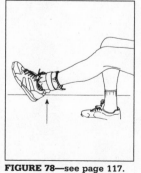

FIGURE 78—see page 117.

FIGURE 83—see page 118.

CHAPTER 15

THE FUTURE

O nce you're involved in some sort of exercise on a regular basis, there are endless possibilities of what you can do. Some good ideas for starting are mentioned here. The important thing is to start. If you become bored, there are many different activities which will keep you fit. Plyometrics (jumping), medicine balls, closed chain exercises, calisthenics, stepping exercises, stretching, various racquet sports, dancing, jogging, swimming, cycling, exercise classes, rowing, mini-trampolines, walking, roller blading, basketball, weight lifting, to name a few.

Choose one or several and mix and match them to suit your particular situation. They can easily be developed into a circuit or circuit-interval training program. The ultimate circuit program *to date* is the Iron(person) Triathlon—try swimming a couple of miles, running a marathon (twenty-six miles), and cap it off with a half a century (fifty miles) bike ride. On second thought, don't try. Instead adjust the activities for the everyday Lazy Person, like most of us. If you're interested in all or some of these activities, there are excellent reference works on "how to" and training routines. The President's Council on Physical Fitness and Sports has a wealth of information for the asking. The address is:

701 Pennsylvania Avenue, N.W.

Suite 250

Washington, D.C. 20004

It's good to set goals for yourself both in how often and how much to exercise. You might start with a goal of how long you walk, say thirty minutes. Then add to that how far you can go in the thirty minutes (in other words, how many miles per hour). You could set a goal of toning up the muscles and shaping your anatomy (use that ultra-sophisticated testing device—the tape measure). Set a goal of weight loss (say hello to Mr. Scale). Or simply "feeling better," having more energy and a zest for life. No matter what the goal, and make sure it's reasonable, you should periodically measure your progress. Go slowly, exercise longer not harder, and watch the changes occur.

Whatever reasons you have to begin exercise, exercise will not be maintained as a regular part of your life unless you derive some pleasure from it. This is difficult to imagine when you begin, but it can happen. You may come to enjoy just the movement of your body itself.

Find activities you *like*. This might be going to the gym and working out while ogling or identifying with the beautiful bodies, bicycling in the outdoors, playing Frisbee with your kids, racquetball or tennis with your friends, or anything else. The key is to find activities that *you enjoy*. Maybe there aren't any now, but if you experiment with enough kinds of physical activity, a miracle might occur and you might find some. Maybe you tried golf once and didn't like it, but have you tried it *lately*? Perhaps your mind set has changed, and you can see it with new eyes.

Or perhaps you can try different activities with your new body. A few months of any kind of exercise may have changed your body enough that things you couldn't do or enjoy before become easier and, dare we say it, fun.

Another key to maintaining an exercise program is to change it. After a few months of any program, vary it, at least slightly. If you've been doing isotonic exercises, change them a little. If you've been lifting weights for your biceps in a straight arc, try turning the weight as you go up. Start out with your palm facing down, and as you bring the weight up, turn your wrist so that the exercise ends with the palm up.

Test out the many variations on each exercise, some with weights, some with tubing, some isometric, and some variations within those for each muscle group the Lazy Person's guide has suggested. Other exercise books contain other variations.

As you try different activities, your aerobic workout may change, too. You may bicycle outside more in the summer, early fall, and late spring, and do more indoor workouts in winter. Tennis can be indoors or out. As you try different approaches to movement, don't be afraid to replace an old standard with a new activity that appeals to you. This will help stay with your exercise program.

Consider approaches you wouldn't have before. Tai Chi may not conform to the description of aerobic exercise, isometric, or isotonic, but in China it's certainly believed to be beneficial to health. If anything, it embodies the isokinetic principles so hard to get without expensive equipment.

How about yoga? Or dance? The trick is to try.

The social aspect of exercise is very important to maintenance. Gyms these days are great places to meet people. Playing tennis or racquetball with a friend adds a new dimension to your relationship and gets both of you to exercise.

Most important is not to become an exercise bore. Your exercise routine may be a topic of conversation in the gym, or with like-minded acquaintances at a cocktail party, but you can also bore people to death with it. If whomever you're talking to takes a sudden interest in the door or his watch, it might be time to change the subject. Be sensitive to ironic or sarcastic comments, and be prepared to drop the exercise topic in favor of Michael Jordan's latest career move.

CHAPTER 16

EXERCISE AND WELLNESS

As we move further and further away from our human origins of hunters and gatherers, we're less and less active. On a worldwide basis, we're spending more and more time in sedentary occupations with little time left over for physical activity. Now while saber-toothed tiger injuries have decreased, there are more chronic degenerative illnesses in all populations.

There seems to be a clear link between exercise and wellness, from improving our heart and lung function to maintaining our immune system, which is under an increasing attack from all sides.

To maintain our cardiovascular health, exercise is necessary. It can reduce blood pressure and body weight. Aerobic exercise helps to control fat and cholesterol in our bodies. Considering that this book is intended for the Lazy Person, a formal exercise program may not be in the cards. It may be that your exercise has to be incorporated into the day's activities. So walk around that office quickly, park at the far end of the lot, take one flight of stairs up and two down, stand up and stretch, and do your isometrics.

The link between exercise and cancer is not clear at present, but there is some evidence that physical activity can help reduce the risk. Certainly, exercise is not a magic bullet to kill cancers, but remaining fit and active along with proper nutrition can only be beneficial. And certainly for those people with cancer, exercise can help to maintain the highest level of function possible as well as giving the person a sense of well-being. These exercises, of course, must be guided by a health team knowledgeable about programs for cancer patients.

While we know there is a relationship between exercise and the immune system, we still have little knowledge of it. Researchers are not yet sure of the net effect, positive or negative. People who regularly exercise to exhaustion and athletes who are overtrained are noted to have a decrease in immune function. On the other hand, those who exercise and increase their aerobic capacity are noted to have an increase in immune function. There are many questions still to be answered on this front.

The last two aspects of exercise and wellness that need to be mentioned are obesity control and mood. While it's difficult to burn calories because of the great amount of exercise which is required to burn just one calorie, exercise helps with fat control. It's not clear whether exercise raises the set point for some time after the workout, or whether there is some mechanism we don't yet understand.

There is a greater willingness and ability to eat properly when exercising, and there is certainly a sense of well-being that accompanies exercise. After a vigorous workout, there is often a mood elevation which raises the spirit and gives some sense of satisfaction having gone through the rigors of exercising.

The last and clearly demonstrable effect of exercise and wellness is the maintenance and development of our musculoskeletal system. Properly conditioned muscles are necessary for good posture, preventing injury to our joints, and in making it easy to go about our daily activities. Osteoporosis, or thinning of the bones, which is very common in women, can be reduced or delayed with proper exercise. The effects of osteoarthritis, the common form of arthritis from which many people suffer, can be lessened with proper exercise to maintain the flexibility of the joint and keep the muscles around it strong.

On the whole, exercise seems to be beneficial to various aspects of the functioning of our bodies. This includes the muscles and bones, the heart and lungs, the immune system, the blood composition, and the frame of mind.

Okay. It's time for us to confess. No matter what impression we tried to give you initially, it does take *some* effort to get fit. But sweating doesn't have to be bad. You can learn to like exercising, if you haven't already. What you can definitely learn to like is the healthier, more active, more attractive you that getting fit will bring. Lazier people than you—trust us, there are some—have said "I think I can, I think I can" and they have. Now it's your turn. We know you can. We know you can.

See you at the gym.